PLANNING A WIC RESEARCH AGENDA

WORKSHOP SUMMARY

Carol West Suitor, Rapporteur

Food and Nutrition Board

INSTITUTE OF MEDICINE
OF THE NATIONAL ACADEMIES

THE NATIONAL ACADEMIES PRESS
Washington, D.C.
www.nap.edu

THE NATIONAL ACADEMIES PRESS 500 Fifth Street, N.W. Washington, DC 20001

NOTICE: The project that is the subject of this report was approved by the Governing Board of the National Research Council, whose members are drawn from the councils of the National Academy of Sciences, the National Academy of Engineering, and the Institute of Medicine.

This study was supported by Contract No. AG-3198-C-10-0004 between the National Academy of Sciences and the U.S. Department of Agriculture. Any opinions, findings, conclusions, or recommendations expressed in this publication are those of the author(s) and do not necessarily reflect the view of the organizations or agencies that provided support for this project.

International Standard Book Number 0-13: 978-0-309-16179-4
International Standard Book Number 0-10: 0-309-16179-4

Additional copies of this report are available from the National Academies Press, 500 Fifth Street, N.W., Lockbox 285, Washington, DC 20055; (800) 624-6242 or (202) 334-3313 (in the Washington metropolitan area); Internet, http://www.nap.edu.

For more information about the Institute of Medicine, visit the IOM home page at: **www.iom.edu.**

Printed in the United States of America

The serpent has been a symbol of long life, healing, and knowledge among almost all cultures and religions since the beginning of recorded history. The serpent adopted as a logotype by the Institute of Medicine is a relief carving from ancient Greece, now held by the Staatliche Museen in Berlin.

Suggested citation: IOM (Institute of Medicine). 2011. *Planning a WIC Research Agenda: Workshop Summary.* Washington, DC: The National Academies Press.

"Knowing is not enough; we must apply.
Willing is not enough; we must do."
—Goethe

INSTITUTE OF MEDICINE
OF THE NATIONAL ACADEMIES

Advising the Nation. Improving Health.

THE NATIONAL ACADEMIES

Advisers to the Nation on Science, Engineering, and Medicine

The **National Academy of Sciences** is a private, nonprofit, self-perpetuating society of distinguished scholars engaged in scientific and engineering research, dedicated to the furtherance of science and technology and to their use for the general welfare. Upon the authority of the charter granted to it by the Congress in 1863, the Academy has a mandate that requires it to advise the federal government on scientific and technical matters. Dr. Ralph J. Cicerone is president of the National Academy of Sciences.

The **National Academy of Engineering** was established in 1964, under the charter of the National Academy of Sciences, as a parallel organization of outstanding engineers. It is autonomous in its administration and in the selection of its members, sharing with the National Academy of Sciences the responsibility for advising the federal government. The National Academy of Engineering also sponsors engineering programs aimed at meeting national needs, encourages education and research, and recognizes the superior achievements of engineers. Dr. Charles M. Vest is president of the National Academy of Engineering.

The **Institute of Medicine** was established in 1970 by the National Academy of Sciences to secure the services of eminent members of appropriate professions in the examination of policy matters pertaining to the health of the public. The Institute acts under the responsibility given to the National Academy of Sciences by its congressional charter to be an adviser to the federal government and, upon its own initiative, to identify issues of medical care, research, and education. Dr. Harvey V. Fineberg is president of the Institute of Medicine.

The **National Research Council** was organized by the National Academy of Sciences in 1916 to associate the broad community of science and technology with the Academy's purposes of furthering knowledge and advising the federal government. Functioning in accordance with general policies determined by the Academy, the Council has become the principal operating agency of both the National Academy of Sciences and the National Academy of Engineering in providing services to the government, the public, and the scientific and engineering communities. The Council is administered jointly by both Academies and the Institute of Medicine. Dr. Ralph J. Cicerone and Dr. Charles M. Vest are chair and vice chair, respectively, of the National Research Council.

www.national-academies.org

PLANNING COMMITTEE FOR WIC RESEARCH NEEDS: A WORKSHOP*

GAIL G. HARRISON (*Chair*), Professor, School of Public Health, and Director, Center for Global and Immigrant Health, University of California, Los Angeles
MAUREEN BLACK, Scholl Family Professor of Pediatrics, University of Maryland, School of Medicine, Baltimore, MD
PATRICIA B. CRAWFORD, Co-Director, Center for Weight and Health and Adjunct Professor, School of Public Health, Department of Nutritional Sciences and Technology, University of California, Berkeley
BARBARA DEVANEY, Senior Vice President and Director, Human Services Research, Mathematica Policy Research, Inc., Princeton, NJ
MIRIAM LABBOK, Professor of the Practice of Public Health, Carolina Global Breastfeeding Institute, Department of Maternal and Child Health, University of North Carolina, Chapel Hill
JACKSON P. SEKHOBO, Director, Evaluation and Analysis Unit, Bureau of Administration and Evaluation, Division of Nutrition, New York State Department of Health, Albany, NY
SHANNON E. WHALEY, Director of Research and Evaluation, Public Health Foundation Enterprise WIC Program, Irwindale, CA

Study Staff

SHEILA MOATS, Study Director
CAROL WEST SUITOR, Consultant and Rapporteur
SAUNDRA LEE, Senior Program Assistant (until October 15, 2010)
ANTON L. BANDY, Financial Associate
GERALDINE KENNEDO, Administrative Assistant
LINDA D. MEYERS, Director, Food and Nutrition Board

---

*Institute of Medicine planning committees are solely responsible for organizing the workshop, identifying topics, and choosing speakers. The responsibility for the published workshop summary rests with the workshop rapporteur and the institution.

Reviewers

This report has been reviewed in draft form by individuals chosen for their diverse perspectives and technical expertise, in accordance with procedures approved by the National Research Council's Report Review Committee. The purpose of this independent review is to provide candid and critical comments that will assist the institution in making its published report as sound as possible and to ensure that the report meets institutional standards for objectivity, evidence, and responsiveness to the study charge. The review comments and draft manuscript remain confidential to protect the integrity of the process. We wish to thank the following individuals for their review of this report:

Janet Currie, Department of Economics, Columbia University
Philip M. Gleason, Senior Fellow, Mathematica Policy Research, Inc.
Julie Reeder, Senior Research Analyst, WIC Program, Oregon Department of Human Services
Jamie S. Stang, Department of Food Science and Nutrition, University of Minnesota School of Public Health

Although the reviewers listed above have provided many constructive comments and suggestions, they did not see the final draft of the report before its release. The review of this report was overseen by **Melvin Worth (retired),** Institute of Medicine. Appointed by the National Research Council he was responsible for making certain that an independent examination of this report was carried out in accordance with institutional procedures and that all review comments were carefully considered. Responsibility for the final content of this report rests entirely with the author and the institution.

Contents

Overview

The time has come to initiate a new program of research on the Special Supplemental Nutrition Program for Women, Infants, and Children (commonly referred to as WIC). WIC is the third-largest food assistance program administered by the U.S. Department of Agriculture (USDA) (USDA/ERS, 2009). The program's scope is large: During the final quarter of fiscal year (FY) 2009, approximately 9.3 million low-income women,[1] infants, and children younger than 5 years who were at nutritional risk received WIC benefits each month. Through federal grants to states, participants receive three types of benefits: (1) a supplemental food package tailored to specific age groups for infants and children and to physiological status for women; (2) nutrition education, including breastfeeding support; and (3) referrals to health services and social services. WIC is available in all 50 states and the District of Columbia, 34 Indian Tribal Organizations, Guam, American Samoa, the Commonwealth Islands of the Northern Marianas, Puerto Rico, and the Virgin Islands. Ninety state agencies administer the program through approximately 2,200 local agencies and 9,000 clinic sites. To cover program costs for FY 2010, Congress appropriated $7.252 billion. Congress also appropriated $15 million for research related to the program for FY 2010, which ended a long period in which there was very little funding for WIC research.

The timing of the funding for WIC research is propitious. In October 2009, USDA issued regulations that made substantial revisions to the WIC food package. These revisions are the first major change in the food pack-

[1]To be categorically eligible, a woman must be pregnant or post partum or be breastfeeding.

age since the program's inception in 1972 (Public Law 92-433, section 17 amendment to the Child Nutrition Act of 1966). The development of the new food package regulations relied heavily on the Institute of Medicine report *WIC Food Packages: Time for a Change* (IOM, 2006). The revisions bring the packages into alignment with the current recommendations from the *Dietary Guidelines for Americans* (HHS/USDA, 2005) for more fruits and vegetables and whole grains. The revisions also place a priority on breastfeeding.

The new funding for WIC research is timely for several additional reasons. Much of the research on the outcomes of WIC participation was conducted at least 20 years ago. For example, the seminal WIC–Medicaid Study sponsored by the Food and Nutrition Service (USDA/FNS, 1990), which used data from the years 1987 and 1988, was published in 1990. Over the intervening years WIC has expanded greatly, Medicaid coverage has increased, large changes have occurred in the racial and ethnic backgrounds and socioeconomic status of WIC participants as well as in public health services, and obesity rates have increased substantially among the general population.

To guide its planning for the use of the $15 million allocated for WIC research, the Food and Nutrition Service of USDA asked the Institute of Medicine to convene an ad hoc committee to plan and conduct a 2-day public workshop on emerging research needs for WIC. As requested, the workshop was planned to include presentations and discussions that would illuminate issues related to future WIC research issues and methodological challenges and solutions as well as the planning of a program of research to determine the effects of WIC on maternal and child health outcomes and costs.

The Food and Nutrition Board of the Institute of Medicine held a workshop called "Health Impacts of WIC—Planning a Research Agenda" on July 20–21, 2010. The workshop agenda appears in Appendix A. The seven planning committee members, who are listed in the front matter of this report, served as moderators for the sessions. The workshop opened with remarks by three key figures in the administration and history of the program. This was followed by nine themed sessions featuring 33 expert researchers from multiple fields of study who gave formal presentations or served as discussants or moderators. Information on these researchers is provided in Appendix B. Each session included a period for discussion that was open to all those in attendance. To prepare for the workshop, presenters were given the following guidance:

1. Considering previous research and research that is currently under way, identify direction(s) for future research related to the session topic.

2. State the rationale and significance of each specified direction for future research.
3. Specify a time frame for proposed study or series of studies.
4. Discuss methodological approaches and challenges.
5. Discuss or suggest potential data sources.

The moderator of each session held a conference call with the presenters and discussants to clarify the five parts of the guidance and to coordinate preparations for the workshop. Presenters were asked not to present a comprehensive review of the published research on a topic. However, each presenter and discussant was asked in advance to identify independently the research topic that he or she thought should receive the highest priority. In advance of the workshop, the discussants were provided with copies of the slides for their session to help them prepare their response to the presentations made during the session. To help prepare for the methodology presentations, the presenters received, in advance, separate sets of slides covering the previous sessions and were asked to comment on methods as appropriate.

From June 11, 2010, through August 2, 2010, the website http://iom.edu/Activities/Nutrition/WICResearchAgenda/2010-JUL-20.aspx was open to receive comments about the workshop and about research needs related to WIC. During the workshop, all attendees were invited to contribute further comments to the website, and presenters and discussants were asked to submit their top three research priorities to the website.

THE WORKSHOP

This report is a summary of the workshop presentations and discussions and has been prepared from workshop transcripts and slides. In some instances, content has been reorganized for greater clarity. Presenters and discussants made specific recommendations or suggestions, as requested. However, none of the statements in this workshop summary, including those made during the closing session (Chapter 10), represent a consensus regarding conclusions or recommendations.

To provide more details about the workshop and its participants, Appendix A contains the workshop agenda, Appendix B contains the biographical sketches of the presenters, Appendix C lists the workshop attendees and their affiliations, and Appendix D identifies acronyms and abbreviations. Appendix E summarizes comments that were posted on the website for the workshop, some of which address points made in response to workshop presentations. Appendix F is an abbreviated compilation of suggested research topics and methods.

REFERENCES

HHS/USDA (U.S. Department of Health and Human Services/U.S. Department of Agriculture). 2005. *Dietary Guidelines for Americans*. 6th ed. Washington, DC: U.S. Government Printing Office. http://www.health.gov/DietaryGuidelines/dga2005/document/ (accessed September 16, 2010).

IOM (Institute of Medicine). 2006. *WIC Food Packages: Time for a Change*. Washington, DC: The National Academies Press.

USDA/ERS (U.S. Department of Agriculture/Economic Research Service). 2009. *Economic Linkages Between the WIC Program and the Farm Sector: Economic Brief Number 12*. Washington, DC: USDA/ERS. http://www.ers.usda.gov/Publications/EB12/EB12.pdf (accessed August 24, 2010).

USDA/FNS (U.S. Department of Agriculture/Food and Nutrition Service). 1990. *The Savings in Medicaid Costs for Newborns and Their Mothers from Prenatal Participation in the WIC Program, Volume 1*. Alexandria, VA: USDA/FNS.

1

Opening Session

This workshop provided the participants with the opportunity to inform the Food and Nutrition Service of the U.S. Department of Agriculture (USDA) about the priorities and needs for research related to the Special Supplemental Nutrition Program for Women, Infants, and Children (commonly called WIC). In her opening remarks, Gail Harrison, chair of the planning committee and workshop moderator, said that the workshop represents an unprecedented opportunity in that USDA currently has some substantial funds to allocate to WIC research—funds that need to be committed rather quickly.

The workshop was organized to cover eight topics:

1. WIC and birth outcomes;
2. WIC and overweight and obesity;
3. WIC and breastfeeding;
4. Food insecurity and hunger;
5. Dietary intake and nutritional status;
6. Nutrition education;
7. Health care and systems costs, benefits, and effectiveness; and
8. The reach of WIC.

Although methodology was discussed in the sessions covering each of these topics, the closing session was planned to include two presentations specifically addressing methodological issues raised during the workshop.

The opening session featured brief presentations from three persons who have played key roles in support of WIC over time: Jay Hirschman, Reverend Douglas Greenaway, and David Page.

PERSPECTIVES FROM THE U.S. DEPARTMENT OF AGRICULTURE

Presenter: Jay Hirschman[1]

WIC was conceived as a national program during the White House Conference on Nutrition in 1969 and was first operated as a pilot program under a different name beginning in 1972. Since then, it has grown to serve more than one-third of all pregnant women, half of all infants, and 30 percent of all children younger than 5 years of age in the United States. Figure 1-1 illustrates the program's steady growth.

Hirschman said that USDA is seeking the best ideas and most important research questions relating to the impacts of WIC in its current form and in potential future forms, being respectful of funding realities regarding benefits. In fiscal year (FY) 2010, WIC received up to $15 million for studies and evaluations, and the President's budget request for FY 2011 asks for a similar amount. These amounts are substantially higher than those received in previous years.

WIC is intended to foster growth and development among those U.S. women, infants, and children with the lowest incomes and greatest need. It does so through a regular supply of nutritious foods, nutrition education, breastfeeding support, and referrals. Over the years, WIC has relied on scientifically based research and evaluations to guide policy development and provide justification for improved program coverage. Nonetheless, because a wide variety of changes have occurred in WIC and in the environment in which WIC operates (see Box 1-1), Hirschman said a new program of research is needed to provide a basis for adapting and improving WIC.

Hirschman asked that all attendees consider the information presented at the workshop and then submit to the workshop website hosted by the Institute of Medicine their recommendations and rationale for three projects that should receive funding priority.

PERSPECTIVES FROM THE NATIONAL WIC ASSOCIATION

Presenter: Reverend Douglas Greenaway

The National WIC Association (NWA) recognizes, Greenaway said, that the scientific evidence supporting the benefits of WIC is outdated; and NWA welcomes the support for WIC research provided by the 111th

[1]Hirschman expressed thanks to Congress; the National WIC Association; the Centers for Disease Control and Prevention; all WIC's partners at the state, territorial, tribal, and local levels; vendors; food manufacturers; and many others for helping make WIC one of the best programs that the nation has to offer.

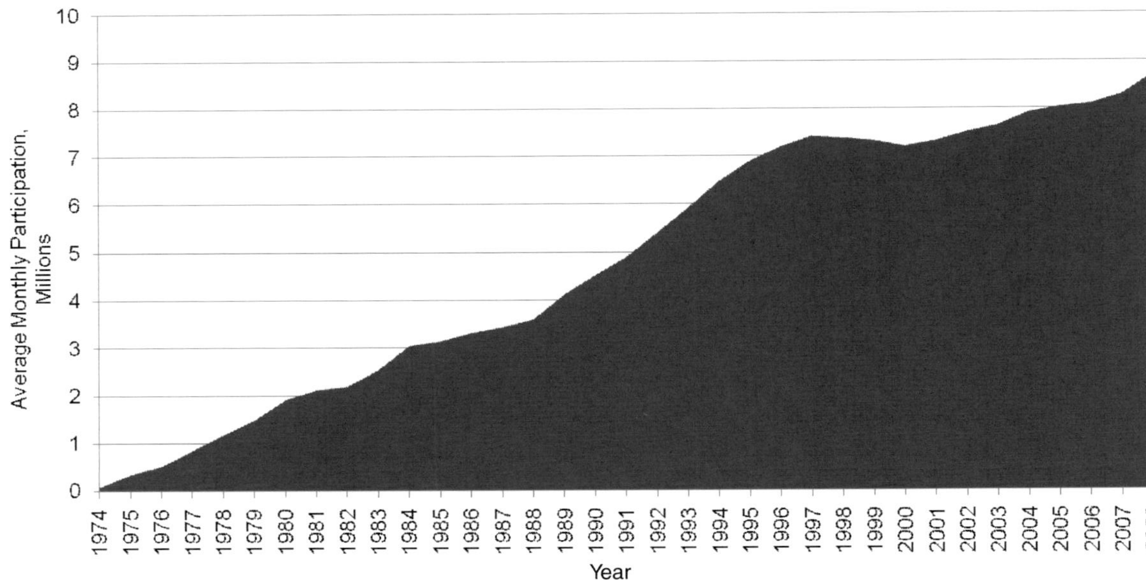

FIGURE 1-1 Average monthly participation in the Special Supplemental Nutrition Program for Women, Infants, and Children, 1974–2009.
SOURCE: Hirschman (2010).

BOX 1-1
Changes in WIC and the Environment in Which WIC Operates

Changes to WIC

- Revised WIC food packages (October 2009)
- Increased size of the participating population
- Full funding (no wait lists)
- Earlier enrollment during pregnancy (now 50 percent enroll during the first trimester) (USDA/FNS, 2006)
- Changed ethnic distribution of the WIC-eligible population (more Hispanics)
- Increased focus on breastfeeding promotion and support (and more funding)
- Increased length of certification period for infants
- Transition from paper vouchers to electronic benefit transfer (EBT) (in process)

Changes to the Environment in Which WIC Operates

- Expansion of other programs—Medicaid and similar programs, State Children's Health Insurance Program (SCHIP), Head Start, Early Head Start, and the Supplemental Nutrition Assistance Program (SNAP)
- The new health care legislation
- A shift in nutrition education from the "traditional medical model" to client-centered, motivational methods
- The economic recession that began in 2007
- New technology
- Changes in the food supply, including expansion of the foods meeting WIC criteria
- Changes in the health risks of the U.S. population (especially increased obesity)
- Development of new growth charts
- Changes in social norms relating to food, nutrition, and eating (including a growing demand for local sustainable foods)

Congress. Greenaway said that the current study of the impact of WIC participation on Medicaid costs will provide valuable cost–benefit data.

NWA's Evaluation Committee has identified the following four research priorities for consideration:

1. *Examine the most effective strategies for WIC to use in support of exclusive breastfeeding and in the promotion of the initiation and duration of breastfeeding. This examination is to include peer counseling services in addition to other breastfeeding support services and strategies that WIC provides.* Despite clear evidence of the health benefits of breastfeeding and improved initiation rates (currently 74 percent), the rates of exclusive breastfeeding drop off quickly, and only 23 percent of infants are breastfed for 12 months.

2. *Identify and assess prevention and intervention strategies that WIC uses to reduce the risk of overweight and obesity, and evaluate their effectiveness.* The President's Task Force Report on Childhood Obesity (White House Task Force on Childhood Obesity, 2010) summarizes evidence that one in five children is overweight or obese before the age of 6 years and that more than half of obese children have become overweight by the age of 2 years.
3. *Examine the modes of nutrition education delivery, evaluate their effectiveness, and identify best practices that can be shared easily.* WIC requires two nutrition education contacts per certification period. The purpose of the contacts is to assist participants in achieving a positive change in dietary and physical activity habits and thereby improving their nutritional status and decreasing their risks of nutrition-related problems.
4. *Evaluate how the recent changes to the WIC food packages have influenced the dietary behaviors of WIC mothers and young children.*

In addition, NWA recommends that the use of functional food additives (such as nucleotides, docosahexaenoic acid, pre-biotics, and pro-biotics) be evaluated to determine potential benefits and drawbacks in foods that are part of the WIC food package. NWA is concerned that such products increase costs and may provide little, if any, benefit.

Anticipated changes in WIC under the Affordable Care Act include the implementation of electronic benefit delivery systems by 2020, the updating of related systems, and the release of health data in more useable formats. Such changes could give WIC the opportunity to examine data collection methods and to determine future data needs and capacities. Improved WIC data collection, in turn, could lead to substantial contributions to the knowledge base of maternal and child health outcomes and costs.

OPENING REMARKS

Presenter: David Paige

Scientific data provided a foundation for WIC and have guided its programmatic decisions. Research has been at the heart of the program. According to Paige, the continuing evolution of the program requires that attention be paid to a new set of research questions and some new approaches. These include consideration of the following:

- Critical periods of discrete risks and varying levels of vulnerability, such as those relating to folic acid deficiency, fetal alcohol syndrome, and infant feeding choices
- Clear definitions of birth outcomes

- The heterogeneity of the obesity problem in terms of its origins, impacts, adaptations, and relationship to the environment
- New factors that may affect breastfeeding initiation, duration, and exclusivity, including the new food packages, personnel (especially peer counselors), mixed rather than unified messages, and the medicalization of breastfeeding
- Additives to infant formula
- Effective targeting of foods to food-insecure families and careful follow-up
- Ways to improve outreach
- Development of an electronic system to exchange key information about the client, aid in the integration of WIC services into the health care system, and reduce client burden

A restructured, reinvigorated, and cost-efficient approach to delivering WIC services would focus on prevention (e.g., trying to make the pregnancy "the best that there is"), integrate WIC into a comprehensive health system, increase partnering with the community, and exploit social networking and other new technologies to enhance nutrition education and give WIC clients a voice in the services they receive.

REFERENCES

Hirschman, J. 2010. *Health impacts of WIC: Planning a WIC research agenda.* Presented at the Institute of Medicine Workshop on Health Impacts of WIC–Planning a Research Agenda, Washington, DC, July 20–21.

USDA/FNS (U.S. Department of Agriculture/Food and Nutrition Service). 2006. *WIC Participant and Program Characteristics 2004.* Alexandria, VA: USDA/FNS. http://www.fns.usda.gov/ora/MENU/Published/WIC/FILES/pc2004.pdf (accessed November 10, 2010).

White House Task Force on Childhood Obesity. 2010. *Solving the Problem of Childhood Obesity Within a Generation.* Washington, DC: White House Task Force on Childhood Obesity. http://www.letsmove.gov/pdf/TaskForce_on_Childhood_Obesity_May2010_FullReport.pdf (accessed September 16, 2010).

2

WIC and Birth Outcomes

During this session, moderated by Gail Harrison, the two presenters (Michael Lu and Theodore Joyce) addressed selected topics related to maternal health and nutrition and birth outcomes, and the two discussants (Marianne Bitler and Patrick Catalano) added clarifying information. Each of them recommended topics for the research agenda for the Supplemental Nutrition Program for Women, Infants, and Children (WIC).

THE ROLE OF PERICONCEPTIONAL NUTRITION

Presenter: Michael Lu

The path toward a healthier population begins with improving periconceptional nutrition, emphasized Lu. The periconceptional period extends from preconception through conception, implantation, placentation, embryogenesis, and organogenesis. These are critical stages that affect both immediate birth outcomes and also the long-term health and development of the child.

Research Background

Increasingly, studies have linked periconceptional nutrition to reproductive outcomes. These outcomes include ovulatory infertility (Botto et al., 2004; Chavarro et al., 2006, 2007a,b,c, 2008a,b), birth defects (Groenen et al., 2004; Krapels et al., 2004; Lumley et al., 2001; Smedts et al., 2008; Velie et al., 1999; Verkleij-Hagoort et al., 2006), spontaneous preterm birth

(Bukowski et al., 2009; Vahratian et al., 2004), preeclampsia (Bodnar et al., 2006; Catov et al., 2007), and infants with low birth weight and who are small for their gestational age (Timmermans et al., 2009). For example, the First and Second Trimester Evaluation of Risk (FASTER) trial found that preconceptional folate supplementation for at least 1 year was associated with a lower risk of spontaneous extreme preterm birth (20–28 weeks) and that the risk was inversely proportional to the duration of preconceptional folate supplementation.

Although the biological mechanisms linking periconceptional nutrition with specific reproductive outcomes are not clearly understood, Lu indicated that some evidence makes connections that are biologically plausible. For example, nutrition plays a role in host susceptibility to infection and inflammation, and these in turn may be related to placental complications. In approximately one-third of the cases of preterm birth, the placental vessels show failure of vascular remodeling, and in 15 to 25 percent they show residual vascular pathology characterized by thrombosis and atherosis (see Figure 2-1).

Lu briefly reviewed evidence of the role of the placenta in fetal programming and future disease risk (see Godfrey, 2002) and noted potential effects of periconceptional nutrition on epigenetic modification (Sinclair et al., 2007; Steegers-Theunissen et al., 2009). In particular, he emphasized periconceptional nutrition as it relates to allostasis and allostatic load. Allostasis refers to the maintenance of stability through change, and allostatic load refers to the cumulative physiological toll from chronic stress. Chronic, repeated stress causes the body to lose its ability for self-regulation (McEwen, 1998). Lu postulated that chronically "bombarding" the body with high-sugar and high-fat diets and with high stress will gradually re-

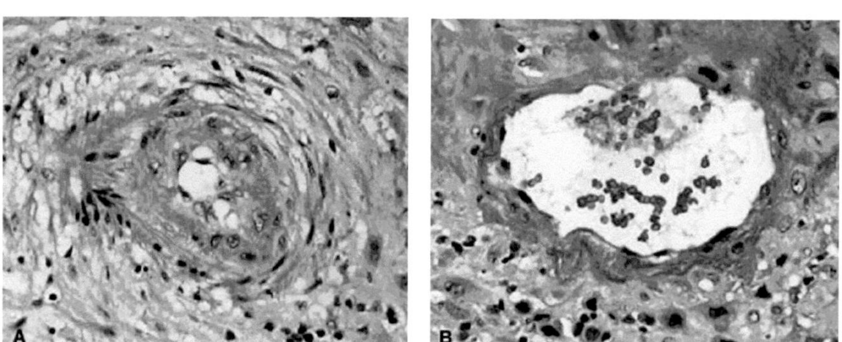

FIGURE 2-1 (A) Spiral artery in a preterm pregnancy; (B) spiral artery in a normal pregnancy.
SOURCE: Salafia and Popek (2008). Reprinted with permission.

duce the body's ability to self-regulate and will damage regulatory systems to the point that fetal programming will be sub-optimal. Lu stated that the interconception period provides a critical window of opportunity to restore allostasis to optimize the woman's health before she becomes pregnant.

Research Proposals

Lu said that the research mentioned above makes it clear that the agenda for WIC research should include studies conducted during interconception in order to address the preconceptional period before a subsequent pregnancy. His three research proposals were:

1. *Observational studies on the effect of interconceptional nutrition on birth and long-term child health outcomes.* These studies should incorporate biomarkers to identify mechanisms and pathways. Consider potential collaboration with the National Children's Study through adjunct studies. Through the provider-based recruitment strategies being used, WIC sites could potentially be valuable for study participant recruitment.
2. *Nutritional intervention studies that begin at interconception.* Prioritize women with previous adverse outcomes and communities with marked nutrition and health disparities. Conduct single nutrient, multi-nutrient, and whole foods supplementation studies. Conduct both efficacy and effectiveness research.
3. *Nutritional research that focuses on women's health before, between, and beyond pregnancy.* Outcomes to consider include metabolic allostasis and allostatic load, postpartum weight retention, and breastfeeding.

In closing, Lu said, "I think it is really time that we put the 'W' back in WIC."

THE IMPACT OF WIC ON BIRTH OUTCOMES

Presenter: Theodore Joyce

Joyce opened by saying that there is relatively weak evidence that WIC protects against adverse birth outcomes. He agreed with Lu that the focus needs to be on maternal health, beginning at preconception. His presentation briefly addressed the level of prenatal intervention that WIC provides and evidence from early studies of WIC, pointed out challenging sources of methodological biases (especially gestational age bias and postpartum bias), and made suggestions for a change in focus.

Level of the Intervention

Given that the average period a pregnant woman is on WIC is 4.5 months, that the average monthly prenatal food voucher is worth approximately $50, and that the marginal propensity to consume[1] is about 20 percent for WIC, Joyce estimated that WIC provides about $45 in extra food consumption for the pregnancy. This amount alone, he argued, cannot explain the very large improvements in birth outcomes associated with WIC participation that have been reported in the literature.

Evidence from Early Experimental Studies

Three early high-quality experimental studies (Klerman et al., 2001; Metcoff et al., 1985; Rush et al., 1980) reported no effect from WIC or nutritional supplementation during pregnancy on birth outcomes, but they are seldom cited. The study by Rush and colleagues even concludes that protein supplementation may be a risk factor for preterm birth.

Sources of Bias

Time-series evidence is inconsistent with large treatment effects. Considering the findings by Devaney et al. (1992) of about a 4 percent difference in low birth weight between WIC participants and nonparticipants on Medicaid, one would expect to see a change in the rate of low birth weight over time. But although WIC enrollment has quadrupled since 1983, there has been no visible effect of WIC enrollment on low birth weight rates (see Figure 2-2). Similarly, there is no visible association between WIC enrollment and singleton preterm birth rates. In a report on preterm birth, the Institute of Medicine (IOM, 2007) concluded that little is known about how to prevent these early births.

A number of studies of low birth weight and preterm birth have used methods that introduce large biases. For example, gestational age bias may arise because women with longer-term pregnancies have more time to enroll in WIC as a prenatal participant. Compared with the women who enroll early, those who enroll late in their pregnancy are more likely to have good birth outcomes simply because the pregnancy went to term (Devaney, 2010). An example of gestational age bias is shown in Figure 2-3. A notable feature of the graph is that the rate of low birth weight decreases dramatically for women who enroll in WIC very late in their pregnancy. Obviously, this improvement in low birth weight rates cannot be attributed to WIC.

---

[1] In this case, the *marginal propensity to consume* assumes that if a person is given a specific amount of money, X percent of it would be spent on *extra* food consumption.

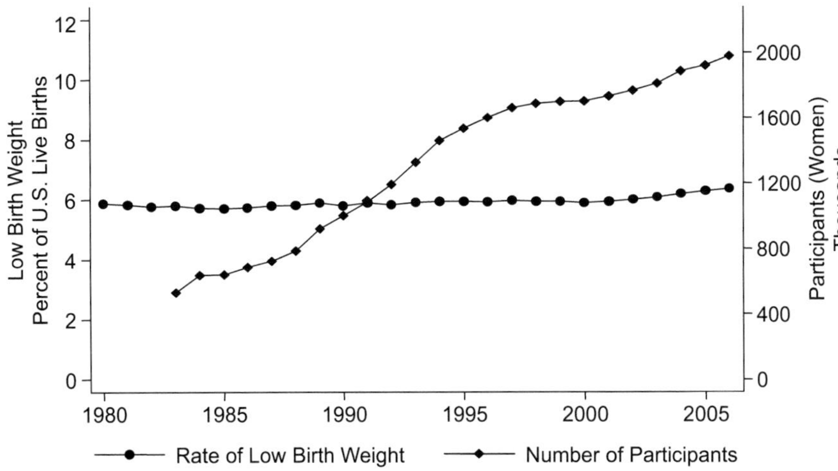

FIGURE 2-2 Rate of low birth weight (singleton births) versus number of WIC participants, United States, 1983–2007.
SOURCE: Joyce (2010), using participation data from Christopher Swann, University of North Carolina at Greensboro (unpublished).

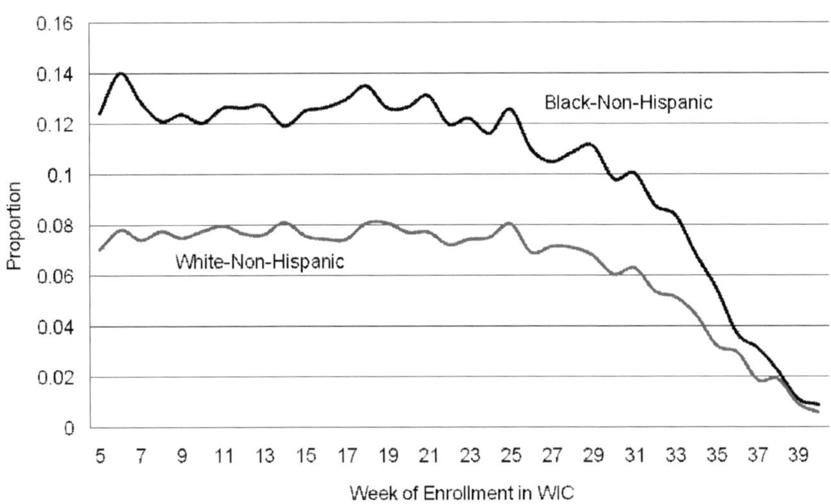

FIGURE 2-3 Rate of low birth weight by race and week of prenatal WIC enrollment (author's tabulations from North Carolina Pregnancy Nutrition Surveillance System, 1996–2003).
SOURCE: Joyce (2010).

Comparing the rate of preterm births for women who enrolled prenatally with those who enrolled post partum may introduce another bias related to the reason for the late enrollment. Data from the North Carolina Pregnancy Surveillance System suggest that postpartum bias occurs when the outcome is preterm birth but not when the outcome is the number of newborns who are small for their gestational age. When prenatal and postnatal enrollees are compared with regard to age, education, ethnic background, participation in Medicaid and food stamps, and prenatal smoking, postpartum bias is evident. That is, the characteristics of the women who enrolled after giving birth are more favorable to good pregnancy outcomes than are the characteristics of the women who enrolled when pregnant.

Changing the Research Focus

The research agenda needs to focus on maternal health and behaviors, Joyce said. Maternal health provides a mechanism by which to improve infant and child health. Among the key factors are preconceptional smoking (rates of which are extremely large for white, non-Hispanic North Carolina WIC participants), obesity (applicable to a large percentage of women of childbearing age), prenatal weight gain (which exceeds Institute of Medicine recommendations for a large proportion of women), and breastfeeding (for which racial and ethnic differences are extremely large). It would be useful to collect data on body mass index whenever a woman visits the WIC office, as well as on blood pressure and low-density lipoproteins, and on hemoglobin A1c for women with diabetes. In the same way that some entities are working to change unhealthful behaviors such as smoking, consider paying women to breastfeed rather than to bottle feed.

Summarizing Thoughts

Joyce concluded his presentation by suggesting that research should move away from a focus on birth outcomes and toward improving maternal health as the means to improve infant health. Low-cost ways of collecting basic health data are needed.

RESPONSE

Discussant: Marianne Bitler

Methodological Issues

Quality of the Evidence

Standards of evidence have become more rigorous over time. Selection bias may explain some of the positive effects that have previously been reported for WIC participation. As an example of selection bias, women who choose to participate in WIC may be more motivated than WIC-eligible non-participants. However, there appears to be little evidence of positive selection for WIC participation when women are drawn from Medicaid samples.

Bitler questioned whether selection bias was sufficient to account for all the differences discussed by Joyce, giving two examples of studies that addressed selection bias carefully. In particular, Hoynes et al. (2010) looked at the roll out of WIC at the county level and demonstrated statistically significant improvements in average birth weight and reductions in low birth weight among WIC participants. Also, Figlio et al. (2009) used tight participant and non-participant comparison groups (based on income close to the threshold for WIC) and found a reduction in low birth weight associated with WIC participation.

Time Series Interpretation

WIC may have different effects for different subgroups. With the expansion of WIC eligibility over time, some of the added participants may benefit less than the original group. This could partially account, for example, for the lack of change in the rate of low birth weights in the time series graph (Figure 2-2) shown by Joyce.

Channels Through Which WIC Works

Progress is needed in understanding the channels through which WIC works. As Joyce explained earlier, the monetary value of the WIC food package is not likely to be enough to explain the positive effects attributed to WIC; but the WIC food package may change the composition of the food consumed by participants. Within the WIC setting, women may already be predisposed to good behavior, and there may be better opportunities to move participants in the right direction.

Research Proposals

Bitler suggested a version of a randomized controlled trial that could be conducted in WIC settings:

1. Identify the domains through which WIC appears to have an effect (e.g., nutritional advice, smoking cessation).
2. Offer competitive grants to clinics to improve along one of the dimensions.
3. Choose clinics that qualify, and randomly assign some of them to be awarded money and some of them not.

Bitler also made data-related suggestions similar to those Joyce had made: (1) find ways to link up Centers for Disease Control and Prevention surveillance data and make it more publicly available, and (2) collect data beyond simply WIC participation and timing of entry in WIC.

Concluding Thoughts

In summary, Bitler concluded that there is compelling evidence that (1) WIC works on some dimensions, (2) the mechanisms by which WIC works need to be understood, (3) randomized designs are needed to help provide this information, and (4) data need to be linked and made more publicly available.

RESPONSE

Discussant: Patrick M. Catalano[2]

A 1990 study (USDA/FNS, 1990) showed that women who participated in WIC during their pregnancies had lower Medicaid costs for themselves and their babies than did women who did not participate. WIC participation was also linked with longer gestation periods, higher birth weights, and lower infant mortality. Many changes have occurred since that study was conducted, however. The nation has experienced an obesity epidemic, for example, and diabetes rates are closely tied to obesity rates. Based on proposed criteria for gestational diabetes, about 16 to 20 percent of U.S. women may now be classified as having gestational diabetes.

Although only one time series shown earlier by Joyce is consistent with the growth in WIC participation—namely, the one depicting the rates of infants born who are small for their gestational age (Figure 2-4), data from Catalano's hospital indicate that the adjusted average birth weight increased by 120 grams from 1975 to 2003. The entire birth weight curve has shifted up, and pregravid maternal obesity is the factor that has the strongest correlation with the change in the birth weight curve.

Although trends in preterm birth have not improved with increased WIC participation (Figure 2-3), a larger proportion of the preterm births are now late preterm births occurring between 34 and 36 weeks of gestation rather than before 34 weeks (Figure 2-5). Much of this change may be related to changes in obstetrical practice (earlier delivery of infants). Furthermore, definitions need to be considered when examining birth weights. For example, the decrease in average birth weight in some studies may be

[2]Because of travel delays, Catalano was unable to hear the preceding presentations. However, he had advance access to Lu's and Joyce's slides.

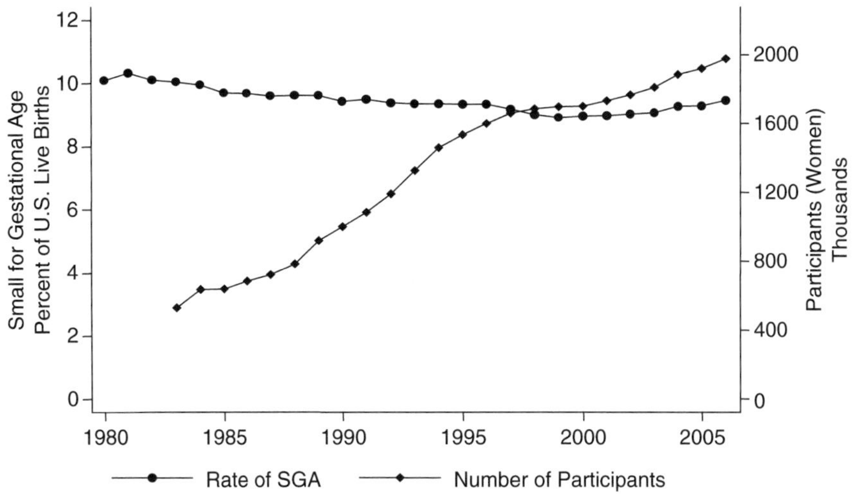

FIGURE 2-4 Rate of small-for-gestational-age births versus number of WIC participants, United States, 1983–2007.
SOURCE: Joyce (2010), using participation data from Christopher Swann, University of North Carolina at Greensboro (unpublished).

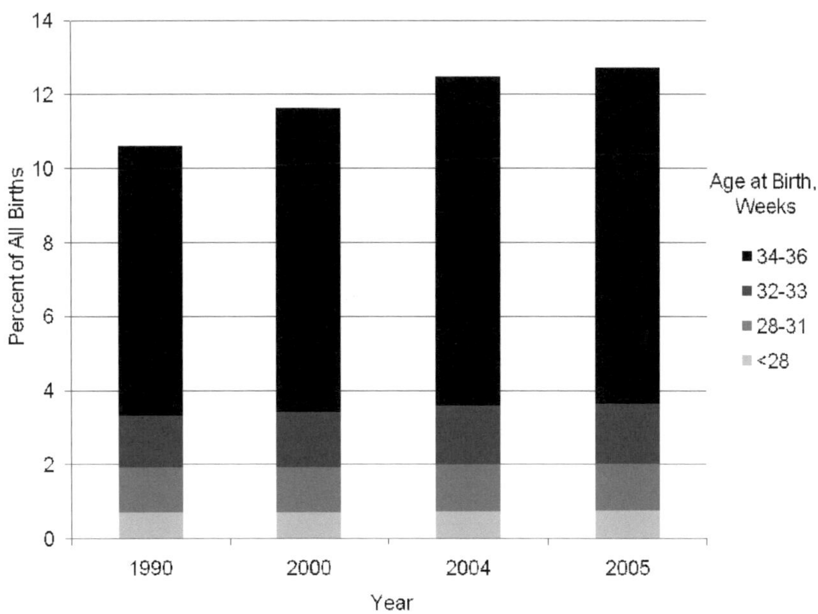

FIGURE 2-5 Distribution of preterm births by gestational age, 1990–2005.
SOURCE: NCHS (2007).

explained by earlier delivery of neonates that are classified as full-term infants.

Catalano said that pregravid weight and weight gain during pregnancy merit attention. Gestational weight gain by underweight women substantially decreases the risk of having an infant that is small for gestational age, but gestational weight gain has little effect on that risk for overweight and obese women. It is worth noting that high gestational weight gain[3] by underweight women is accompanied by a 50 percent increase in the newborn's fat mass, but the long-term significance of that fat gain is unknown. Nonetheless, Catalano said, pregravid body mass index is the strongest predictor of adiposity of the newborn at birth, followed by gestational age and gestational weight gain; it also is the strongest predictor of the percentage of body fat at age 8 years.

Research Proposals

The dollar amount available for WIC research is relatively small. Hence, Catalano believes the research question or questions need to be specific and directed toward the health of the mother. Most importantly, addressing the health of the pregnancy should begin *before* pregnancy, if possible, but at the very least early in pregnancy, and it should continue through the postpartum (interconceptional) period. Pregnancy offers a teachable moment. Accordingly, Catalano stressed that the research needs to be multispecialty, including pediatricians, obstetricians, and allied health professionals such as nutritionists and physical educators, with emphasis placed on factors related to lifestyle, such as diet, exercise, and smoking cessation.

GROUP DISCUSSION

Moderator: Gail G. Harrison

The session's presenters, as well as David Paige, participated in the brief discussion and raised the following points:

- Paige suggested that to understand the impact of WIC participation, we may need new metrics for identifying risks. Low birth weight (≤2,500 g), for example, is not a sensitive tool to measure impact. Preterm birth, about which very little is known, does not indicate either low birth weight or intrauterine growth restriction. One needs to distinguish long-term from short-term fetal growth

[3]In excess of Institute of Medicine recommendations (>20 kg).

restriction. By contrast, congenital anomaly indicates a problem very early in pregnancy and is a major cause of death.

- Joyce used preterm birth as an example in his presentation because it was a key measure of effect in early reports of the effectiveness of WIC and also because preterm birth is closely linked with low birth weight and extremely closely linked with very low birth weight.
- Paige and Lu emphasized that WIC needs to be better integrated with the health care system to achieve a more comprehensive, effective, and targeted delivery system.
- Catalano reemphasized the need to determine appropriate sizes for neonates born to women of widely different body mass index and to identify the gestational weight gain associated with appropriate fetal growth.

SUMMARY OF SUGGESTED RESEARCH TOPICS

The research suggestions made during this session focused on the mother's health and behaviors rather than on the infant. These suggestions included observational studies and nutritional interventions especially during the interconceptual period and an approach for conducting randomized controlled trials in the clinic setting to test carefully selected interventions. It was pointed out that there is a need for data collection that goes beyond WIC participation status and time of enrollment and for improved data linkages and public access to the data. Also, it was suggested that collaboration with the National Children's Study may be possible through adjunct studies.

REFERENCES

Bodnar, L. M., G. Tang, R. B. Ness, G. Harger, and J. M. Roberts. 2006. Periconceptional multivitamin use reduces the risk of preeclampsia. *American Journal of Epidemiology* 164(5):470–477.

Botto, L. D., R. S. Olney, and J. D. Erickson. 2004. Vitamin supplements and the risk for congenital anomalies other than neural tube defects. *American Journal of Medical Genetics Part C: Seminars in Medical Genetics* 125C(1):12–21.

Bukowski, R., F. D. Malone, F. T. Porter, D. A. Nyberg, C. H. Comstock, G. D. Hankins, K. Eddleman, S. J. Gross, L. Dugoff, S. D. Craigo, I. E. Timor-Tritsch, S. R. Carr, H. M. Wolfe, and M. E. D'Alton. 2009. Preconceptional folate supplementation and the risk of spontaneous preterm birth: A cohort study. *PLoS Medicine* 6(5):e1000061.

Catov, J. M., L. M. Bodnar, R. B. Ness, N. Markovic, and J. M. Roberts. 2007. Association of periconceptional multivitamin use and risk of preterm or small-for-gestational-age births. *American Journal of Epidemiology* 166(3):296–303.

Chavarro, J. E., J. W. Rich-Edwards, B. A. Rosner, and W. C. Willett. 2006. Iron intake and risk of ovulatory infertility. *Obstetrics and Gynecology* 108(5):1145–1152.

Chavarro, J. E., J. W. Rich-Edwards, B. A. Rosner, and W. C. Willett. 2007a. A prospective study of dairy foods intake and anovulatory infertility. *Human Reproduction* 22(5):1340–1347.

Chavarro, J. E., J. W. Rich-Edwards, B. A. Rosner, and W. C. Willett. 2007b. Diet and lifestyle in the prevention of ovulatory disorder infertility. *Obstetrics and Gynecology* 110(5):1050–1058.

Chavarro, J. E., J. W. Rich-Edwards, B. A. Rosner, and W. C. Willett. 2007c. Dietary fatty acid intakes and the risk of ovulatory infertility. *American Journal of Clinical Nutrition* 85(1):231–237.

Chavarro, J. E., J. W. Rich-Edwards, B. A. Rosner, and W. C. Willett. 2008a. Use of multivitamins, intake of B vitamins, and risk of ovulatory infertility. *Fertility and Sterility* 89(3):668–676.

Chavarro, J. E., J. W. Rich-Edwards, B. A. Rosner, and W. C. Willett. 2008b. Protein intake and ovulatory infertility. *American Journal of Obstetrics and Gynecology* 198(2):210.e1–210.e7.

Devaney, B. 2010. WIC Turns 35: Program Effectiveness and Future Directions. In *Cost Effective Programs in Children's First Decade: A Human Capital Integration*, edited by A. J. Reynolds, A. Rolnick, M. M. Englund, and J. Temple. New York: Cambridge University Press.

Devaney, B., L. Bilheimer, and J. Schore. 1992. Medicaid costs and birth outcomes: The effects of prenatal WIC participation and the use of prenatal care. *Journal of Policy Analysis and Management* 11(4):573–592.

Figlio, D., S. Hamersma, and J. Roth. 2009. Does prenatal WIC participation improve birth outcomes? New evidence from Florida. *Journal of Public Economics* 93(1-2):235–245.

Godfrey, K. M. 2002. The role of the placenta in fetal programming—A review. *Placenta* 23(Suppl. A):S20–27.

Groenen, P. M., I. A. van Rooij, P. G. Peer, M. C. Ocke, G. A. Zielhuis, and R. P. Steegers-Theunissen. 2004. Low maternal dietary intakes of iron, magnesium, and niacin are associated with spina bifida in the offspring. *Journal of Nutrition* 134(6):1516–1522.

Hoynes, H., M. Page, and A.H. Stevens (article under review). 2010. Can targeted transfers improve birth outcomes? Evidence from the introduction of the WIC program.

IOM (Institute of Medicine). 2007. *Preterm Birth: Causes, Consequences, and Prevention.* Washington, DC: The National Academies Press.

Joyce, T. 2010. *The impact of WIC on birth outcomes.* Presentation at the IOM workshop, Health Impacts—Planning a WIC Research Agenda. Washington, DC, July 20–21.

Klerman, L. V., S. L. Ramey, R. L. Goldenberg, S. Marbury, J. Hou, and S. P. Cliver. 2001. A randomized trial of augmented prenatal care for multiple-risk, Medicaid-eligible African American women. *American Journal of Public Health* 91(1):105–111.

Krapels, I. P., I. A. van Rooij, M. C. Ocke, C. E. West, C. M. van der Horst, and R. P. Steegers-Theunissen. 2004. Maternal nutritional status and the risk for orofacial cleft offspring in humans. *Journal of Nutrition* 134(11):3106–3113.

Lumley, J., L. Watson, M. Watson, and C. Bower. 2001. Periconceptional supplementation with folate and/or multivitamins for preventing neural tube defects. *Cochrane Database of Systematic Reviews* (3):CD001056.

McEwen, B. S. 1998. Protective and damaging effects of stress mediators. *New England Journal of Medicine* 338(3):171–179.

Metcoff, J., P. Costiloe, W. M. Crosby, S. Dutta, H. H. Sandstead, D. Milne, C. E. Bodwell, and S. H. Majors. 1985. Effect of food supplementation (WIC) during pregnancy on birth weight. *American Journal of Clinical Nutrition* 41(5):933–947.

NCHS (National Center for Health Statistics). 2007. Births: Final data for 2005. *National Vital Statistics Report* 56(6):1–104. http://www.cdc.gov/nchs/data/nvsr/nvsr56/nvsr56_06.pdf (accessed September 16, 2010).

Rush, D., Z. Stein, and M. Susser. 1980. A randomized controlled trial of prenatal nutritional supplementation in New York City. *Pediatrics* 65(4):683–697.

Salafia, C. M., and E. J. Popek. 2008. Plancental development and early pregnancy pathology. In *Global Library of Women's Medicine*, edited by J. J. Sciarra. http://www.glowm.com/index.html?p=glowm.cml/section_view&articleid=150 (accessed September 16, 2010).

Sinclair, K. D., C. Allegrucci, R. Singh, D. S. Gardner, S. Sebastian, J. Bispham, A. Thurston, J. F. Huntley, W. D. Rees, C. A. Maloney, R. G. Lea, J. Craigon, T. G. McEvoy, and L. E. Young. 2007. DNA methylation, insulin resistance, and blood pressure in offspring determined by maternal periconceptional B vitamin and methionine status. *Proceedings of the National Academy of Sciences USA* 104(49):19351–19356.

Smedts, H. P., M. Rakhshandehroo, A. C. Verkleij-Hagoort, J. H. de Vries, J. Ottenkamp, E. A. Steegers, and R. P. Steegers-Theunissen. 2008. Maternal intake of fat, riboflavin and nicotinamide and the risk of having offspring with congenital heart defects. *European Journal of Nutrition* 47(7):357–365.

Steegers-Theunissen, R. P., S. A. Obermann-Borst, D. Kremer, J. Lindemans, C. Siebel, E. A. Steegers, P. E. Slagboom, and B. T. Heijmans. 2009. Periconceptional maternal folic acid use of 400 microg per day is related to increased methylation of the IGF2 gene in the very young child. *PLoS One* 4(11):e7845.

Timmermans, S., V. W. Jaddoe, A. Hofman, R. P. Steegers-Theunissen, and E. A. Steegers. 2009. Periconception folic acid supplementation, fetal growth and the risks of low birth weight and preterm birth: The Generation R Study. *British Journal of Nutrition* 102(5):777–785.

USDA/FNS (U.S. Department of Agriculture/Food and Nutrition Service). 1990. *The Savings in Medicaid Costs for Newborns and Their Mothers from Prenatal Participation in the WIC Program, Volume 1*. Alexandria, Virginia: USDA/FNS.

Vahratian, A., A. M. Siega-Riz, D. A. Savitz, and J. M. Thorp, Jr. 2004. Multivitamin use and the risk of preterm birth. *American Journal of Epidemiology* 160(9):886–892.

Velie, E. M., G. Block, G. M. Shaw, S. J. Samuels, D. M. Schaffer, and M. Kulldorff. 1999. Maternal supplemental and dietary zinc intake and the occurrence of neural tube defects in California. *American Journal of Epidemiology* 150(6):605–616.

Verkleij-Hagoort, A. C., J. H. de Vries, N. T. Ursem, R. de Jonge, W. C. Hop, and R. P. Steegers-Theunissen. 2006. Dietary intake of B-vitamins in mothers born a child with a congenital heart defect. *European Journal of Nutrition* 45(8):478–486.

3

WIC and Obesity

The focus of this session, moderated by Patricia Crawford, was research on how the Special Supplemental Nutrition Program for Women, Infants, and Children (WIC) could have an impact on behaviors that contribute to childhood obesity. The two presenters (Robert Whitaker and Elsie Taveras) identified possible behavioral intervention targets and discussed different aspects of suggested research methods. The discussant (Sara Benjamin Neelon) raised a number of questions about the selection of behavioral intervention targets. The session did not address research on efforts by WIC to address obesity.

RESEARCH PROPOSALS FOR OBESITY PREVENTION AMONG CHILDREN IN WIC

Presenter: Robert C. Whitaker

Whitaker covered four key research findings and their implications for future research. In addition, he mentioned structural constraints in WIC that limit potential research designs, and he proposed a research agenda and a potential staged research design.

Key Research Findings

Four research findings have implications for the WIC research agenda, Whitaker said. They are:

1. *Participation in WIC is not associated with obesity.* Because of this, exposure to WIC *alone* is unlikely to either cause or protect against obesity, and body mass index (BMI) will not be a useful measure of a primary outcome (Hofferth and Curtin, 2005; Ploeg et al., 2008; Rose et al., 2006).
2. *The prevalence of obesity in WIC children no longer seems to be increasing.* Because favorable secular trends are likely to continue among WIC and non-WIC children, careful attention must be given to the control condition when designing studies (Sharma et al., 2009).
3. *Within the WIC income range, higher income is associated with a greater rather than a lower prevalence of obesity.* Thus qualitative studies are needed to examine the complex relationship between childhood obesity and household behaviors and resources (Anderson and Whitaker, 2010; Karp et al., 2005; Whitaker and Orzol, 2006).
4. *Successful prevention or treatment interventions in young children require parental involvement.* Therefore, parents should be the primary targets of interventions to prevent childhood obesity (Epstein et al., 1994; Golan and Crow, 2004; Golan et al., 2006).

Structural Constraints

Because WIC currently has no waivers or wait lists, it is challenging to develop feasible random assignment designs. Interventions must work within WIC's three core functions: the provision of the food package, nutrition education, and referrals.

Proposed Research Agenda

Whitaker's research proposal is given below, followed by his criteria for selecting target behaviors.

Proposal

Develop and test the impact of a coordinated communication strategy among WIC, Head Start, and pediatricians on changing behaviors that help prevent obesity among children 12 to 60 months of age.

Target Behaviors

The target behaviors selected should meet three criteria, namely, that the behavior (1) has an effect on energy balance or weight, (2) is

BOX 3-1
Menu of Target Behaviors

1. Decrease portion sizes.
2. Increase the frequency of family meals.
3. Limit sweetened beverages.
4. Increase outdoor play time with parents.
5. Decrease time spent watching television and on computers.
6. Increase sleep duration.

unlikely to do harm, and (3) has a favorable effect on non-obesity outcomes, such as improving social well-being. The lack-of-harm criterion is especially important when the evidence of benefit is weak. The effect on outcomes other than obesity may provide the key to engaging parents and partners.

Whitaker's menu for target behaviors appears in Box 3-1. According to Whitaker, behavior numbers 5 and 6 in this box, which have consistently been associated with a lower prevalence of obesity, also may lead to improvements in children's moods and decreased aggressive behaviors—possible outcomes that may engage parents.

Potential Staged Design

Whitaker proposed a multistage research design in which each stage informs the next (Box 3-2). The first four stages entail the development of

BOX 3-2
Potential Multistage Research Design

Development of the Communication Strategy
1. Conduct formative qualitative research.
2. Help messengers be healthy through staff wellness programs.
3. Convene messengers to help them understand shared goals and challenges.
4. Develop communication tools, and qualitatively assess both the messages and the medium with messengers and parents.

Testing of the Communication Strategy
5. Pilot-test the communication strategy and the outcome measures.
6. Conduct a controlled impact evaluation.

a communications strategy, which is tested in the fifth and sixth stages. The first stage is the most important. It includes framing messages on behavioral targets and reconciling differences between the frames[1] held by those delivering and those receiving the messages. A key part of the fourth stage is a qualitative assessment of how well both the messages and the medium resonate with the messengers and the parents.

The pilot test (stage 5) would focus on assessing the acceptability, feasibility, and fidelity of delivering the message. If the results of the pilot test are unfavorable, stage 6 would not go forward. If the results of the first five stages warrant a controlled evaluation of the impact of the communication strategy (stage 6), this stage would probably be conducted using a group- or community-randomized design that compares traditional WIC services with WIC services plus an enhanced coordinated communication strategy. The primary outcome should be the target behavior or behaviors. A process and cost evaluation would be an important element of the study in order to determine how to implement the intervention on a larger scale and then to sustain it.

Closing Comments

In closing, Whitaker emphasized that any interventions that are part of the research agenda should target behaviors rather than BMI, that the target behaviors must matter to the WIC partners and to the parents, and that qualitative research is more important and feasible than quantitative research in the WIC setting.

RESEARCH OPPORTUNITIES IN WIC FOR CHILDHOOD OBESITY

Presenter: Elsie M. Taveras[2]

Although the most recent statistics show that the prevalence of childhood obesity has reached a plateau, the prevalence is still high, and obesity is affecting even the nation's youngest children. In 2007–2008, the prevalence of high weight for recumbent length among U.S. children from birth to 2 years of age was 9.5 percent (Ogden et al., 2010), where "high" is defined as weights at or above the 95th percentile of the Centers for Disease Control and Prevention (CDC) growth charts (Kuczmarski et al., 2000). The prevalence of obesity varied by racial and ethnic background,

---

[1]The term *frames* refers to people's perceptions and the meaning that people attribute to objects, events, and behaviors. Frames are likely to differ among WIC staff and WIC partners, such as pediatricians and parents.

[2]Taveras' participation was via conference call, with slides shown on site.

BOX 3-3
Proposed Targets for Behavioral Counseling—Prenatal to Early Childhood

- Gestational weight gain (Oken et al., 2006) and gestational diabetes
- Maternal smoking during pregnancy (Oken et al., 2006)
- Rapid infant weight gain (Taveras et al., 2009)
- Breastfeeding promotion (Taveras et al., 2004)
- Sleep duration and quality (Taveras et al., 2008)
- Television viewing (Taveras et al., 2007) and television sets in bedroom
- Improved responsiveness to infant hunger and satiety cues (Hodges et al., 2008)
- Parental feeding practices, eating in the absence of hunger (Birch and Fisher, 1998; Birch et al., 2003; Taveras et al., 2006a)
- Portion sizes (Fisher et al., 2008)
- Fast food intake (Taveras et al., 2006b)
- Sugar-sweetened beverages (James and Kerr, 2005; Wang et al., 2009)
- Physical activity participation (Gooze et al., 2010; Strong et al., 2005; Tobias et al., 2010)

ranging from 8.7 for non-Hispanic white to 12.5 for Hispanic girls and boys (Ogden et al., 2010). Severe obesity (BMI $\geq$35 kg/m^2) was especially high for Black and Hispanic boys and for Black girls 2 to 19 years of age (Wang et al., 2010).

Relevant Research Findings

Box 3-3 offers a list of proposed targets for behavioral counseling and key references that provide the basis for the inclusion of those targets on the list. Racial and ethnic differences are present in all the early life risk factors for childhood obesity, with children who belong to racial or ethnic minority groups being affected disproportionately. Clearly, prevention must start early, and preventive interventions should be based on the best available evidence for the highest risk populations. WIC fits well with the effort to prevent obesity because of the population groups covered, the structure for screening nutritional status, the nutrition education provided, and the referrals for needed health and social services.

Proposed Research Agenda

Taveras proposed the following study: Develop and test the impact of coordinated surveillance and communication strategies among

1. WIC providers and obstetricians on promoting healthful behaviors during pregnancy to prevent childhood obesity and improve maternal health; and
2. WIC providers, home visitation programs, child care providers, and pediatricians on changing behaviors to help prevent excess weight gain among infants from birth to 12 months.

The targets of intervention during pregnancy would be maternal prepregnancy BMI, excessive gestational weight gain, maternal smoking, and gestational diabetes. The interventions would occur mainly during the inter-pregnancy interval. Taveras called for improving the surveillance of obesity-related risk factors; coordinated referrals and communication strategies; and improvements in parents' ability to handle infant feeding, sleep, and media exposure. A very important communication goal would be to counter the myth that the pregnant woman needs to "eat for two."

The targets of intervention during infancy would be excessive infant weight gain; breastfeeding initiation, continuation, and exclusivity; responsive feeding; portion sizes of bottles and solid food containers; outdoor physical activity; limiting television viewing and televisions in bedrooms; and improving sleep quality and duration. Taveras called for improved surveillance of infant weight gain using the CDC growth charts in combination with the identification of children at high risk of rapid growth and coordinated communication strategies to counter the myth that "bigger is better." Other possible tactics involve education and support that would be directed mainly toward feeding practices and the promotion of physical activity and healthful sleep.

Possible Methodology for Impact Evaluation

Taveras supported the multistage design approach presented by Whitaker and focused on two possible evaluation methods: quasi-experiments and cluster-randomized controlled trials.

Quasi-Experiments

Quasi-experiments, as described by Gortmaker (2004), can have all the attributes of a randomized controlled trial, including pretest and posttest data. The key difference is the lack of random assignment to intervention and control groups. The success of the method depends on appropriate selection of the control sample (e.g., through propensity matching; see Chapter 10). Quasi-experiments make it possible to study programs and policies that are innovative, expensive, and difficult to implement.

Cluster-Randomized Controlled Trials

Cluster-randomized controlled trials are studies in which groups (clusters) are randomized rather than individuals. This method is useful when the intervention is applied to an entire group. Because of the randomization, such trials have better internal validity than quasi-experimental studies. They also allow the study of interventions that cannot be directed toward selected individuals. However, the design and analysis of cluster-randomized controlled trials are complex, the required sample sizes are large, the cost is high, and the long time it takes to obtain study results may preclude rapid evaluations of innovations.

Concluding Comments

Taveras said that WIC can play a substantial role in efforts to prevent childhood obesity during pregnancy, infancy, and early childhood—especially when WIC works in collaboration with partners such as obstetricians, home visitation programs, child care providers, and pediatricians. She concluded that those determining the research agenda should consider innovative study designs and methods as a way of overcoming the barriers to wide-scale intervention testing in WIC.

RESPONSE

Discussant: Sara Benjamin Neelon

Questions Triggered by the Obesity Session Presentations

Benjamin Neelon asked all those present to consider the presentations by Whitaker and Taveras and think about four questions, and she provided her own responses, as follows:

1. *What is WIC already doing and already doing well to prevent childhood obesity?*
   Response: Screening and measuring growth, addressing competing issues within families.
2. *What can WIC do to include more obesity prevention within its current structure?*
   Response: Target various family members and caregivers, not just the mother.
3. *Are there missed opportunities for obesity prevention within WIC?*
   Response: Reaching women during interconceptional periods, engaging fathers and partners.

4. *Where does obesity prevention rank among other behavioral targets within WIC? How would you prioritize obesity prevention when you consider other health concerns?*
   Response: None provided.

Benjamin Neelon also asked attendees to consider behavioral targets according to three different considerations: (1) those that have the greatest effect on obesity prevention, (2) those that WIC is in a good position to address, and (3) those that are or should be integral to the mission of WIC. Some behavioral targets may move WIC nutritionists beyond their training and comfort zone. With these points in mind, Benjamin Neelon highlighted those behavioral intervention targets that she considered to be more promising—that is, the ones for which WIC could have a greater impact (see bolded items in Box 3-4).

Concluding Comments

According to Benjamin Neelon, WIC can play a substantial role in obesity prevention, although it cannot provide the entire answer. WIC needs to engage collaborative partners. Target behaviors must matter to partners and caregivers and must extend beyond weight and obesity. The research design should compare WIC to an enhanced form of WIC. Most importantly, a combination of qualitative and quantitative formative processes and impact evaluation will be needed to assess the effectiveness of new measures.

BOX 3-4
Behavioral Intervention Targets[a]

Pregnancy	Infancy	Early Childhood
Excess weight gain	Excess weight gain	Sweetened beverages
Smoking	Breastfeeding	**Family meals**
Pre-pregnancy BMI	Portion sizes	**Portion sizes**
Gestational diabetes	**Responsive feeding**	**Play/physical activity**
	Play/physical activity	**Screen time**
	TV viewing/TV bedroom	**Sleep quality/duration**
	Sleep quality/duration	

[a]Bold font indicates the targets for which WIC could have a greater impact.

GROUP DISCUSSION

Moderator: Patricia B. Crawford

The following topics were addressed during the discussion period:

- Methods: Considerable evidence shows that quasi-experimental designs such as regression discontinuity and propensity scoring place large demands on the sample size, often requiring sample sizes much larger than those needed for randomized controlled trials (RCTs). When RCTs are feasible, they may be relatively simple and straightforward.
- Healthy Habits for Life kits and the Around Food Insecurity program: These products of a partnership between the National WIC Association and the Sesame Workshop include evaluation components, and they tie in with suggestions for behavior change made during this session.
- Efforts to encourage appropriate infant feeding (exclusive, long-term breastfeeding): These efforts tie together behaviors related to maternal health (postpartum fat loss) and infant health.
- The screening component of WIC: (1) The use of the new World Health Organization growth charts results in identifying overweight children earlier than with the CDC growth charts. (2) Crowded living conditions can lead to positive responses to questions such as, "Is there a TV in the room in which your child sleeps?"
- Formative research related to obesity prevention: This approach has value for 1-year-old children as well as for the older ones.

SUMMARY OF SUGGESTED RESEARCH TOPICS

The research proposals made during this session focused on developing and testing strategies to change behaviors linked with excess weight among infants and young children. Emphasis was placed on collaboration with a range of partners. The method proposed here would involve a multistage research design that would be used to identify target behaviors that matter to partners and caregivers and that extend beyond weight and obesity. The design would also help determine effective ways to address those behaviors. Both qualitative and quantitative research designs will be needed.

REFERENCES

Anderson, S. E., and R. C. Whitaker. 2010. Household routines and obesity in US preschool-aged children. *Pediatrics* 125(3):420–428.

Birch, L. L., and J. O. Fisher. 1998. Development of eating behaviors among children and adolescents. *Pediatrics* 101(3 II Suppl.):539–549.

Birch, L. L., J. O. Fisher, and K. K. Davison. 2003. Learning to overeat: Maternal use of restrictive feeding practices promotes girls' eating in the absence of hunger. *American Journal of Clinical Nutrition* 78(2):215–220.

Epstein, L. H., A. Valoski, R. R. Wing, and J. McCurley. 1994. Ten-year outcomes of behavioral family-based treatment for childhood obesity. *Health Psychology* 13(5):373–383.

Fisher, J. O., N. F. Butte, P. M. Mendoza, T. A. Wilson, E. A. Hodges, K. C. Reidy, and D. Deming. 2008. Overestimation of infant and toddler energy intake by 24-h recall compared with weighed food records. *American Journal of Clinical Nutrition* 88(2):407–415.

Golan, M., and S. Crow. 2004. Parents are key players in the prevention and treatment of weight-related problems. *Nutrition Reviews* 62(1):39–50.

Golan, M., V. Kaufman, and D. R. Shahar. 2006. Childhood obesity treatment: Targeting parents exclusively v. parents and children. *British Journal of Nutrition* 95(5):1008–1015.

Gooze, R. A., C. C. Hughes, D. M. Finkelstein, and R. C. Whitaker. 2010. Reaching staff, parents, and community partners to prevent childhood obesity in Head Start, 2008. *Preventing Chronic Disease* 7(3):A54.

Gortmaker, S. L. 2004. *Scenario 2: Prevention of childhood obesity.* Paper presented at the May 4–5, 2004, Workshop on Research Designs for Complex, Multi-level Health Interventions and Programs, Bethesda, MD. http://obssr.od.nih.gov/news_and_events/conferences_and_workshops/FY_2004/complex_interventions.aspx#dates (accessed September 7, 2010).

Hodges, E. A., S. O. Hughes, J. Hopkinson, and J. O. Fisher. 2008. Maternal decisions about the initiation and termination of infant feeding. *Appetite* 50(2-3):333–339.

Hofferth, S. L., and S. Curtin. 2005. Poverty, food programs, and childhood obesity. *Journal of Policy Analysis and Management* 24(4):703–726.

James, J., and D. Kerr. 2005. Prevention of childhood obesity by reducing soft drinks. *International Journal of Obesity* 29(Suppl. 2):S54–S57.

Karp, R. J., C. Cheng, and A. F. Meyers. 2005. The appearance of discretionary income: Influence on the prevalence of under- and over-nutrition. *International Journal of Health Inequities* 4:10.

Kuczmarski, R. J., C. L. Ogden, L. M. Grummer-Strawn, K. M. Flegal, S. S. Guo, R. Wei, Z. Mei, L. R. Curtin, A. F. Roche, and C. L. Johnson. 2000. CDC growth charts: United States. *Advance Data from Vital and Health Statistics* 314:1–27. http://www.cdc.gov/nchs/data/ad/ad314.pdf (accessed September 24, 2010).

Ogden, C. L., M. D. Carroll, L. R. Curtin, M. M. Lamb, and K. M. Flegal. 2010. Prevalence of high body mass index in US children and adolescents, 2007–2008. *Journal of the American Medical Association* 303(3):242–249.

Oken, E., Y. Ning, S. L. Rifas-Shiman, J. S. Radesky, J. W. Rich-Edwards, and M. W. Gillman. 2006. Associations of physical activity and inactivity before and during pregnancy with glucose tolerance. *Obstetrics and Gynecology* 108(5):1200–1207.

Ploeg, M. V., L. Mancino, B. H. Lin, and J. Guthrie. 2008. US food assistance programs and trends in children's weight. *International Journal of Pediatric Obesity* 3(1):22–30.

Rose, D., J. N. Bodor, and M. Chilton. 2006. Has the WIC incentive to formula-feed led to an increase in overweight children? *Journal of Nutrition* 136(4):1086–1090.

Sharma, A. J., L. M. Grummer-Strawn, K. Dalenius, D. Galuska, M. Anandappa, E. Borland, H. Mackintosh, and R. Smith. 2009. Obesity prevalence among low-income, preschool-aged children—United States, 1998–2008. *Morbidity and Mortality Weekly Report* 58(28):769–773.

Strong, W. B., R. M. Malina, C. J. Blimkie, S. R. Daniels, R. K. Dishman, B. Gutin, A. C. Hergenroeder, A. Must, P. A. Nixon, J. M. Pivarnik, T. Rowland, S. Trost, and F. Trudeau. 2005. Evidence based physical activity for school-age youth. *Journal of Pediatrics* 146(6):732–737.

Taveras, E. M., K. S. Scanlon, L. Birch, S. L. Rifas-Shiman, J. W. Rich-Edwards, and M. W. Gillman. 2004. Association of breastfeeding with maternal control of infant feeding at age 1 year. *Pediatrics* 114(5):e577–e583.

Taveras, E. M., S. L. Rifas-Shiman, K. S. Scanlon, L. M. Grummer-Strawn, B. Sherry, and M. W. Gillman. 2006a. To what extent is the protective effect of breastfeeding on future overweight explained by decreased maternal feeding restriction? *Pediatrics* 118(6): 2341–2348.

Taveras, E. M., T. J. Sandora, M. C. Shih, D. Ross-Degnan, D. A. Goldmann, and M. W. Gillman. 2006b. The association of television and video viewing with fast food intake by preschool-age children. *Obesity* 14(11):2034–2041.

Taveras, E. M., A. E. Field, C. S. Berkey, S. L. Rifas-Shiman, A. L. Frazier, G. A. Colditz, and M. W. Gillman. 2007. Longitudinal relationship between television viewing and leisure-time physical activity during adolescence. *Pediatrics* 119(2):e314–e319.

Taveras, E. M., S. L. Rifas-Shiman, E. Oken, E. P. Gunderson, and M. W. Gillman. 2008. Short sleep duration in infancy and risk of childhood overweight. *Archives of Pediatrics and Adolescent Medicine* 162(4):305–311.

Taveras, E. M., S. L. Rifas-Shiman, M. B. Belfort, K. P. Kleinman, E. Oken, and M. W. Gillman. 2009. Weight status in the first 6 months of life and obesity at 3 years of age. *Pediatrics* 123(4):1177–1183.

Tobias, D. K., C. Zhang, R. M. van Dam, K. Bowers, and F. B. Hu. 2010. Physical activity before and during pregnancy and risk of gestational diabetes mellitus: A meta-analysis. *Diabetes Care*. (Electronically published September 27, 2010).

Wang, Y. C., D. S. Ludwig, et al. 2009. Impact of change in sweetened caloric beverage consumption on energy intake among children and adolescents. *Archives of Pediatrics and Adolescent Medicine* 163(4):336–343.

Wang, Y. C., S. L. Gortmaker, and E. M. Taveras. 2010. Trends and racial/ethnic disparities in severe obesity among US children and adolescents, 1976–2006. *International Journal of Pediatric Obesity*. (Electronically published March 18, 2010).

Whitaker, R. C., and S. M. Orzol. 2006. Obesity among US urban preschool children: Relationships to race, ethnicity, and socioeconomic status. *Archives of Pediatrics and Adolescent Medicine* 160(6):578–584.

4

Research Needed to Improve Breastfeeding Protection, Promotion, and Support Within WIC

OPENING STATEMENT

Moderator: Miriam Labbok

Moderator Miriam Labbok opened the session with a series of slides covering research on the ways in which breastfeeding supports both maternal and infant health, the many adverse effects of *any* formula use (also called lack of breastfeeding), trends in the rate of breastfeeding initiation by the Special Supplemental Nutrition Program for Women, Infants, and Children (WIC) participation status, and WIC participants' much lower rates of exclusive breastfeeding at 3 and 6 months[1] when compared with other WIC-eligible women and with non-eligible women, along with a list of areas where research is needed (Box 4-1). She emphasized the inverted pressure to formula-feed that is related to the formula provided by WIC food packages for infants whose mothers choose not to breastfeed exclusively or partially. During the session, the presenters (Karen Bonuck, Maya Bunik, and Cynthia Howard) focused on different aspects of breastfeeding research and provided suggestions related to surveillance, breastfeeding research involving the WIC food packages, staffing issues (especially peer counseling), and potential research designs. Discussant Larry Grummer-Strawn focused on research related to staffing for breastfeeding support.

[1]The American Academy of Pediatrics recommends that infants be exclusively breastfed for a minimum of 4 months but preferably 6 months (AAP, 2009).

BOX 4-1
Areas Where Breastfeeding Research Is Needed

- Protection
  - Artificially inverted economic pressures related to formula use
  - States' dependency on formula rebates
- Promotion
  - New WIC food package for women who breastfeed exclusively: content, presentation, promotion, and implementation
  - Timing and location of contact
  - Continuity of care
- Support
  - Messaging and how WIC is understood by clients
  - Peer counselors (versus lactation consultants versus other): training, time available, skills for support, and cost-effectiveness
  - Lactation consultants: sufficiency of numbers and availability
- Impact of formula feeding on health

A WIC AGENDA FOR BREASTFEEDING-PROMOTION RESEARCH

Presenter: Karen Bonuck

Lessons from Previous Research

Bonuck began by highlighting lessons for WIC that she had gleaned from a 2008 review by the U.S. Preventive Services Task Force (USPSTF, 2008) of the effects of breastfeeding interventions on initiation, duration, and exclusivity of breastfeeding. Those lessons include:

1. Study quality matters.
2. The continuity of care (breastfeeding interventions) over the prenatal and postnatal periods matters.
3. The focus should be on exclusive breastfeeding rather than *any* breastfeeding.
4. The effects of professional and lay support need to be compared.

Based on preliminary evidence from an ongoing study by her group, Bonuck identified a number of key elements of successful interventions to support breastfeeding:

- Women need information and support across care settings, over time, and in a convenient manner. Information and support are needed as part of prenatal care, during WIC visits, in the hospital, and at home.
- Rapport between the mother and the support person is a key factor determining the effectiveness of support, especially in assisting with such skills as latching on and positioning. Adequate time must be allowed to establish rapport, and cultural matching may be helpful for basic lactation support.
- In-person care reduces the risk of such problems as dehydration and calorie deprivation in the infant, engorgement and mastitis in the mother, and the cessation of breastfeeding for the dyad. Phone calls, pamphlets, and videos should serve as adjuncts to rather than substitutions for face-to-face support.
- Establishing links among health professionals leads to a recognition of the value of breastfeeding support.

Figure 4-1, taken from the WIC Breastfeeding Peer Counseling Study Final Implementation Report (USDA/FNS, 2010), shows the various locations where peer counseling occurs. It illustrates the need to take into

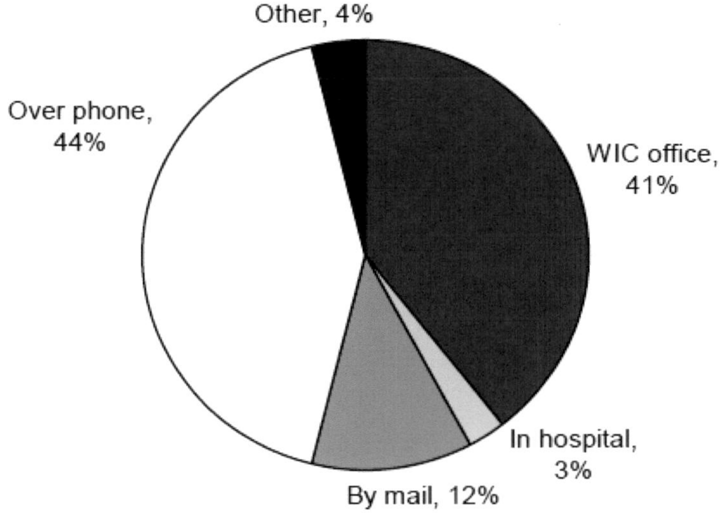

FIGURE 4-1 Location of contacts between WIC participants and peer counselors, fiscal year 2009 (n = 36 local WIC agencies, missing responses from 4).
SOURCE: USDA/FNS (2010).

account the above considerations regarding the location and timing of contacts between WIC participants and peer counselors. It is worth noting that a sizable percentage of WIC agencies prohibit peer counselors from providing guidance in the hospital or in the home, or both.

Challenges in Breastfeeding Support Research

The interpretation of studies of interventions intended to support breastfeeding (e.g., Gross et al., 2009; Olson et al., 2010) is often limited by a lack of data on breastfeeding intensity and sometimes by a lack of data on one or more of the following: actual client contacts, contacts outside of the home, duration of the contact, and problems solved and techniques used to solve them.

Research Suggestions

Based on recommendations from Chapman and Perez-Escamilla (2009), Bonuck provided the following suggestions for national breastfeeding surveillance:

- Use standardized breastfeeding definitions: consider definitions from the Infant Feeding Practices Study II.
- Reduce recall periods to obtain accurate information on the intensity of breastfeeding.
- Collect data on relevant covariates.

Among the key covariates for studies of breastfeeding are prenatal breastfeeding intentions, past breastfeeding history/experience, early hospital experience, reasons for the feeding choice, and the WIC food package the mother has chosen. In addition, it would be useful to collect information on maternal and infant health outcomes, such as the body mass index of the mother and infant and, for the mother, data on cardiovascular disease and diabetes.

BREASTFEEDING ISSUES IN WIC PARTICIPANTS: FOCUS ON SUPPLEMENTATION AND STAFFING ISSUES

Presenter: Maya Bunik

In this presentation, Bunik summarized her perspective on general issues related to breastfeeding research in WIC, identified several attitudes that may interfere with breastfeeding, listed potential study questions, and briefly addressed methods and two types of intervention studies.

General Issues with Breastfeeding Research in WIC

Based on a review of selected studies related to breastfeeding in WIC, Bunik offered the following conclusions:

- There is no need for another cross-sectional survey study on breastfeeding.
- WIC sites vary widely in the way they deliver services.
- The U.S. Department of Agriculture (USDA) does not allow randomization involving the food package.
- Peer counselors seem to be the focus of funding.

Bunik added that WIC agencies need to partner with expert researchers when conducting studies, and WIC staff need time to enter data and develop meaningful databases.

Attitudes That May Interfere with Breastfeeding

According to Bunik, one of the biggest barriers for a mother may be the perception that her milk is insufficient for her infant. Combination feeding may be viewed as offering the infant "the best of both," and there may be little recognition of the impact of supplementing mother's milk with formula (Bunik et al., 2010). Many low-income women are concerned about pain and consider formula feeding to be an easy alternative (Alexander et al., 2010; Bunik et al., 2010). In the Latino culture, the reasons that women give for choosing combination feeding include the pain from breastfeeding, the modesty required in public places, and the need to return to work; parents and grandparents may give strong messages about cultural beliefs (Bunik et al., 2006); and the decision to formula feed may not be viewed with regret.

Study Questions

Bunik offered two sets of study questions for the research agenda.

1. The questions arising from the regulation that specifies that breastfeeding women receive no formula in the first month post partum are:

    - What are the rates in areas that truly practice this policy?
    - How universally is the policy enforced?
    - What is the role of the peer counselor in supporting and reporting on this?

- Are there practices that couple with this policy to make it more effective (e.g., prenatal class, peer counselors, evaluation by an International Board Certified Lactation Consultant (IBCLC), breast pump access)?

2. The questions relating to the numbers and types of core WIC staff members, how they are used, and relationships among them are:

   - Which staff member schedules the "first visit," and how is it done?
   - What WIC staff combinations offer the best outcomes for the breastfeeding dyad?
   - How often is an IBCLC on site?
   - Are WIC staff members empowered enough to "not give out formula"?
   - How do mothers get help early in the breastfeeding experience?
   - Is there communication with the hospital or primary care site?

Research Considerations

Bunik briefly addressed possible research designs, listed in Box 4-2, and then ended her presentation with two suggestions for studying interventions that combine a continuum of care with incentives:

1. Implement a series of prenatal sessions that provides preventive planning (among suggested topics were the possibilities of experiencing pain, barriers during the hospital stay, the need for access to early postpartum help for breastfeeding, and issues of unnecessary supplementation); and provide a blanket or a "hooter hider" as an incentive for attending the sessions.
2. For mothers who choose to breastfeed their newborns, provide no formula in the first month, but offer an early visit and an incentive of diapers to those who have continued to breastfeed at 1 month post partum.

PERSPECTIVES

Presenter: Cynthia R. Howard

Relevant Research Findings

Howard began her presentation by pointing out that research on awareness of and attitudes toward the breastfeeding food package is outdated.

BOX 4-2
Possible Research Designs

- *Randomization by unit, for example, by WIC site or state* Use intraclass correlation coefficient to adjust for this type of randomization.
- *Staggered intervention with each unit as its own control* Use an interrupted time series.
- *Delayed treatment design* Start the intervention at one site, compare to another site that does not have the intervention, and then eventually provide the intervention at the second site as well.

SOURCE: Szilagyi (2010).

The previous package was not seen as valuable, whereas the formula package was seen as very valuable (Holmes et al., 2009; Murimi et al., 2010). Understanding is limited regarding the difference in the health benefits from exclusive breastfeeding and mixed feeding (Bunik et al., 2006; Holmes et al., 2009; Li et al., 2007; Vaaler et al., 2010). Barriers to breastfeeding include concerns about breastfeeding in public (even at home, depending on the household), the lack of availability of breast pumps, the difficulty of pumping, and the transition to work or school (Holmes et al., 2009).

When WIC participants are compared with non-participating WIC eligible women, the rates of exclusive breastfeeding are lower at 4 and 6 months among the WIC participants (Jacknowitz et al., 2007). Moreover, some investigators have found earlier entry into WIC to be associated with lower breastfeeding rates (Gross et al., 2009; Ziol-Guest and Hernandez, 2010). Other investigators (Bunik et al., 2009, Chatterji and Brooks-Gunn, 2004; Joyce et al., 2008; Yun et al., 2010) have reported non-significant or positive effects of WIC participation on breastfeeding outcomes. The conflicting data emphasize the importance of selecting an appropriate control group and gathering data regarding the mother's infant feeding intentions when she enters the program.

Two Cochrane Reviews[2] have addressed breastfeeding and provide information that may help in considering the WIC research agenda. The reviews found:

[2]Systematic reviews that address a clearly formulated question concerning primary research in health care or health policy (Cochrane Reviews, 2010).

1. Needs-based, one-to-one, informal education or support sessions, delivered either (1) before or (2) before and after the birth by a trained breastfeeding professional or peer counselor, were the most effective intervention for promoting breastfeeding initiation among women of different ethnic backgrounds and feeding intentions (Dyson et al., 2005).
2. Trials of breastfeeding support for mothers should consider the timing and delivery of support interventions and the relative effectiveness of intervention components, and they should also report women's views (Britton et al., 2007).

Suggested Research Priorities

Howard addressed research priorities in two topic areas: (1) the effects of the new food package, and (2) the effects of peer counseling. Studies related to the new food package would address breastfeeding initiation, exclusivity (use of the no-formula option), and duration of breastfeeding. Howard provided further detail on the proposed study to examine the effects of peer counseling on breastfeeding and other health outcomes:

- Test components of peer counseling implemented by WIC agencies with high-performing programs, prioritizing exclusive breastfeeding and giving attention to ethnic background, race, and acculturation.
- Test interventions that are feasible, replicable in many setting, and affordable, such as staffing and the supervision of peer counselors; the role of the WIC retailer in facilitating community partnerships; tools to facilitate referrals to WIC from medical care settings and social service agencies; and hospital rounding and collaborations.
- Examine breastfeeding initiation, exclusivity, and duration as major outcomes, but also consider the introduction of solid food and of cow milk, maternal stress and self-confidence, parenting, and family diet.
- Include a qualitative component to assess participant experiences, identify helpful aspects of the intervention, and help guide future processes and policies.

RESPONSE

Discussant: Larry M. Grummer-Strawn

In his response, Grummer-Strawn first introduced key breastfeeding initiatives in WIC and a few related research questions. His major focus, however, was on peer counseling—the topic that was emphasized by the three presenters.

Overview of Key Breastfeeding Initiatives in WIC

The five key breastfeeding initiatives in WIC are: (1) mass media campaigns, (2) WIC food package changes, (3) breast pump distribution, (4) staff training (e.g., "Grow and Glow"), and (5) state incentives. Grummer-Strawn identified one research question related to each initiative:

1. *Mass media* What messages actually motivate behavior change with regard to breastfeeding?
2. *Food packages* What are the effects of the changes in the food packages on breastfeeding rates, especially the rate of exclusive breastfeeding?
3. *Breast pump distribution* Does breast pump distribution increase breastfeeding duration by enabling women to return to work or school, or does it reduce breastfeeding by mechanizing the process, as suggested earlier in the session?
4. *Staff training* Does general training of *all* WIC staff about breastfeeding make enough of a difference in breastfeeding rates to make it worth the additional cost?
5. *State incentives* Do financial incentives to states that provide more money for improvements resulting from breastfeeding promotion in WIC lead to changes in the planning and implementation of programs? Furthermore, what effects do the infant formula rebates have on program decisions?

Research Related to Staffing for Breastfeeding Support

Grummer-Strawn's number one research priority was stronger effectiveness studies of peer counseling within WIC. Funding for peer counseling has grown to $80 million, but, as noted by earlier presenters, the U.S. Preventive Services Task Force found inconclusive evidence of its effectiveness, and there is limited information on the aspects that can improve effectiveness. Such research needs to examine the effects of peer counseling on breastfeeding rates for the entire clinic, not just for the women who choose to use a peer counselor. Moreover, studies need to examine the cost-effectiveness of peer counseling relative to other interventions.

The focus of the research, Grummer-Strawn said, should be on the following components of peer counseling support:

- *Peer counseling training*: What competencies are needed?
- *The role of peer counselors*: Breastfeeding advocates, or supporters of all infant feeding decisions
- *Peer counseling contacts*: Relative importance of prenatal and postpartum contacts, number needed, duration, and type
- *Cultural competency*: Matching of peer counselors with clients, structure in different communities, reaching women who do not want peer counselors
- *Roles of lactation consultants*: Supervision versus individual support, ratio of clients to lactation consultants, relationship to peer counselors
- *Relationship of peer counseling to medical care*: Connections with other providers and care sites, including in-hospital contacts and information flow

Study Design

Although very large sample sizes would be required in ecologic quasi-experimental studies, gathering information on the wide variety of ways in which peer counseling is implemented across the nation would make it possible to examine the differences in the impacts of the various sorts of programs. Given the long list of questions about different aspects of peer counseling, Grummer-Strawn argued for less emphasis on causality (that is, on group-randomized controlled trials, which can answer only one question at a time) and more on plausibility (relative effectiveness of different kinds of programs).

GROUP DISCUSSION

Moderator: Miriam Labbok

Presenters and many attendees participated in a discussion that covered the following topics:

- *Data quality* The collection of accurate data on breastfeeding poses a number of challenges:
    - o Exclusivity is determined from self-report and is more accurate if the question is asked about breastfeeding that day or at some time close to that day. Acceptance of the exclusive breastfeeding package does not mean that the mother is not obtaining formula from other sources (e.g., using manufacturers' coupons to buy formula). The mother's concern about answers that could change the mother-infant dyad's WIC

food packages could contribute to biased responses. Answers obtained at different times from the same mother may be inconsistent.

- o Data are complicated in that the data must be collected longitudinally about a behavior that is changing over time.
- o Local agencies collect little data that are relevant to the impact of peer counseling.
- o Quality control is difficult to implement because tens of thousands of clerks across the nation collect, record, and process data for WIC.
- o Since WIC clinics are not set up to conduct research, researchers need to find an approach that allows a study to benefit the participating clinics or their clients, such as including money for WIC staff in the research budget.

- *Access to data* Not all investigators have access to the data that are collected, because data sharing requires the Health Insurance Portability and Accountability Act (HIPAA) rules be followed.
- *Collaboration* Considering that Medicaid covers the health care of many WIC families and that Medicaid has periodic contact with its clients, beneficial collaborations between WIC and Medicaid could include studies regarding the setting of reimbursement rates for specific services and studies regarding outreach. Data sharing between Medicaid and WIC could also be very valuable. Preliminary data suggest that collaboration is the weakest aspect of the Loving Support Peer Counseling Program,[3] which is currently being evaluated. On the other hand, several workshop attendees encouraged a concerted effort to stay away from collaborations with the formula industry.
- *Preliminary findings* According to Pat Gradziel,[4] with the introduction of the new food package in the California state WIC program, the rate of exclusive breastfeeding jumped upward, the rate of partial breastfeeding decreased substantially, and these changes have persisted. Bonuck's study has found that the trimester of entry into WIC is positively associated with the initiation and duration of breastfeeding but that the effects differ for first births versus higher-order births.
- *Baby Friendly Hospital Initiative (BFHI)* Dr. Labbok reported that research she had done with Eugene Declercq demonstrated positive benefits on breastfeeding may result even if not all 10 steps to suc-

[3]Funded through the Food and Nutrition Service of the U.S. Department of Agriculture.
[4]A workshop attendee who contributed to the discussion.

cessful breastfeeding cited by the BFHI are in place; implementation need not lead to increased costs.

One suggestion for improving the monitoring and surveillance of programs was to identify sentinel programs across the nation and support their efforts to improve the WIC electronic data. Income tiering (looking at incomes at different percentages [e.g., 25, 50, 75, 100, up to 185 percent] of the U.S. Poverty Income Guidelines) is a valuable approach when examining covariates in studies.

SUMMARY OF SUGGESTED RESEARCH TOPICS

The research suggestions made during this session focused mainly on the study of support services for breastfeeding, especially research related to staffing (e.g., roles of peer counselors and IBCLCs, where and when they provide care, and their collaboration with a variety of other care providers) and on the study of breastfeeding incentives and changes in the food packages for the mother-infant dyad. Considerable attention was given to research methods, including the need for (1) improved data collection, quality, and access; (2) feasible experimental designs that give careful attention to the selection of appropriate control groups; and (3) qualitative components of studies to gather data for guiding future efforts and for assessing the relative effectiveness of different kinds of programs.

REFERENCES

AAP (American Academy of Pediatrics). 2009. *Pediatric Nutrition Handbook*, 6th ed. Elk Grove Village, IL: American Academy of Pediatrics.

Alexander, A., D. Dowling, and L. Furman. 2010. What do pregnant low-income women say about breastfeeding? *Breastfeeding Medicine* 5(1):17–23.

Britton, C., F. M. McCormick, M. J. Renfrew, A. Wade, and S. E. King. 2007. Support for breastfeeding mothers. *Cochrane Database of Systematic Reviews*(1):CD001141.

Bunik, M., L. Clark, L. M. Zimmer, L. M. Jimenez, M. E. O'Connor, L. A. Crane, and A. Kempe. 2006. Early infant feeding decisions in low-income Latinas. *Breastfeeding Medicine* 1(4):225–235.

Bunik, M., N. F. Krebs, B. Beaty, M. McClatchey, and D. L. Olds. 2009. Breastfeeding and WIC enrollment in the nurse family partnership program. *Breastfeeding Medicine* 4(3):145–149.

Bunik, M., P. Shobe, M. E. O'Connor, B. Beaty, S. Langendoerfer, L. Crane, and A. Kempe. 2010. Are 2 weeks of daily breastfeeding support insufficient to overcome the influences of formula? *Academic Pediatrics* 10(1):21–28.

Chapman, D. J., and R. Perez-Escamilla. 2009. US national breastfeeding monitoring and surveillance: Current status and recommendations. *Journal of Human Lactation* 25(2): 139–150.

Chatterji, P., and J. Brooks-Gunn. 2004. WIC participation, breastfeeding practices, and well-child care among unmarried, low-income mothers. *American Journal of Public Health* 94(8):1324–1327.

Cochrane Reviews. 2010. *What Are Cochrane Reviews?* Oxford, UK: The Cochrane Collaboration. http://www.cochrane.org/cochrane-reviews (accessed October 15, 2010).

Dyson, L., F. McCormick, and M. J. Renfrew. 2005. Interventions for promoting the initiation of breastfeeding. *Cochrane Database of Systematic Reviews* (2):CD001688.

Gross, S. M., A. K. Resnik, C. Cross-Barnet, J. P. Nanda, M. Augustyn, and D. M. Paige. 2009. The differential impact of WIC peer counseling programs on breastfeeding initiation across the state of Maryland. *Journal of Human Lactation* 25(4):435–443.

Holmes, A. V., N. P. Chin, J. Kaczorowski, and C. R. Howard. 2009. A barrier to exclusive breastfeeding for WIC enrollees: Limited use of exclusive breastfeeding food package for mothers. *Breastfeeding Medicine* 4(1):25–30.

Jacknowitz, A., D. Novillo, and L. Tiehen. 2007. Special Supplemental Nutrition Program for Women, Infants, and Children and infant feeding practices. *Pediatrics* 119(2):281–289.

Joyce, T., A. Racine, and C. Yunzal-Butler. 2008. Reassessing the WIC effect: Evidence from the Pregnancy Nutrition Surveillance System. *Journal of Policy Analysis and Management* 27(2):277–303.

Li, R., V. J. Rock, and L. Grummer-Strawn. 2007. Changes in public attitudes toward breastfeeding in the United States, 1999–2003. *Journal of the American Dietetic Association* 107(1):122–127.

Murimi, M., C. M. Dodge, J. Pope, and D. Erickson. 2010. Factors that influence breastfeeding decisions among Special Supplemental Nutrition Program for Women, Infants, and Children participants from Central Louisiana. *Journal of the American Dietetic Association* 110(4):624–627.

Olson, B. H., S. J. Haider, L. Vangjel, T. A. Bolton, and J. G. Gold. 2010. A quasi-experimental evaluation of a breastfeeding support program for low income women in Michigan. *Maternal and Child Health Journal* 14(1):86–93.

Szilagyi, P. G. 2010. *Crossing the Abyss: From Research to Dissemination/Implementation to Better Health.* http://www.research-practice.org/pdfs/ConferencePresentations/Szilagyi_From_Research _to_Dossemination__Implementation.pdf (accessed September 16, 2010).

USDA/FNS (U.S. Department of Agriculture/Food and Nutrition Service). 2010. *WIC Breastfeeding Peer Counseling Study Final Implementation Report.* Alexandria, VA: USDA/FNS. http://www.fns.usda.gov/ora/menu/published/WIC/FILES/WICPeerCounseling.pdf (accessed September 7, 2010).

USPSTF (U.S. Preventive Services Task Force). 2008. Primary care interventions to promote breastfeeding: U.S. Preventive Services Task Force recommendation statement. *Annals of Internal Medicine* 149(8):560–564.

Vaaler, M. L., J. Stagg, S. E. Parks, T. Erickson, and B. C. Castrucci. 2010. Breast-feeding attitudes and behavior among WIC mothers in Texas. *Journal of Nutrition Education and Behavior* 42(3 Suppl.):S30–S38.

Yun, S., Q. Liu, K. Mertzlufft, C. Kruse, M. White, P. Fuller, and B. P. Zhu. 2010. Evaluation of the Missouri WIC (Special Supplemental Nutrition Program for Women, Infants, and Children) breast-feeding peer counselling programme. *Public Health Nutrition* 13(2):229–237.

Ziol-Guest, K. M., and D. C. Hernandez. 2010. First- and second-trimester WIC participation is associated with lower rates of breastfeeding and early introduction of cow's milk during infancy. *Journal of the American Dietetic Association* 110(5):702–709.

5

Food Insecurity and Hunger

The focus of this session, moderated by Maureen Black, was on research into the interrelationships among food insecurity, the Special Supplemental Nutrition Program for Women, Infants, and Children (WIC), and various health outcomes. *Food insecurity* is defined as "limited or uncertain availability of nutritionally adequate and safe foods or uncertain ability to acquire acceptable foods in socially acceptable ways." *Hunger* (another term used in the following presentations) is defined as the "uneasy or painful sensation caused by a lack of food; the recurrent and involuntary lack of access to food" (Anderson, 1990, pp. 1575–1576). Presenters John Cook and Edward Frongillo each provided background for their research suggestions. Discussant James Weill highlighted some of those suggestions while making a case for emphasizing WIC as a program designed to reduce food insecurity.

FUTURE DIRECTIONS FOR WIC RESEARCH FROM A FOOD SECURITY PERSPECTIVE

Presenter: John T. Cook

Future Context and Environment

To help set the stage for his remarks on a WIC research agenda, Cook identified factors that may influence food security over the coming years. One of the most important factors, according to Cook, will be whether the United States ever develops a meaningful response to global climate change.

Probably the second most important will be whether the United States ever develops a meaningful energy policy. Other factors will include the extent of the economic recovery, the extent of unemployment, the degree to which national food system reforms occur (which relates to obesity), the extent to which global food production responds to demand, and the implementation of health care reform in the United States.

From 1999 until 2007, as can be seen in Figure 5-1, the proportion of U.S. households that were food insecure remained fairly stable, as did the racial and ethnic differences in the level of food insecurity. However, the proportion of food-insecure households increased substantially between 2007 and 2008, the first year of the great economic recession. During that year, the estimated number of children younger than 5 years of age living in food-insecure households increased from 3.54 million to 4.85 million (17.1 percent to 23.1 percent, respectively, of all U.S. children under 5 years). Unemployment was one of the major factors underlying this increase.

In view of the earlier session on obesity, Cook briefly mentioned reviews of the associations between food insecurity and obesity in children and said that findings from the studies have been mixed. He noted that the prevalence of obesity in children of ages 2 years and older essentially leveled off from 2004 to 2008.

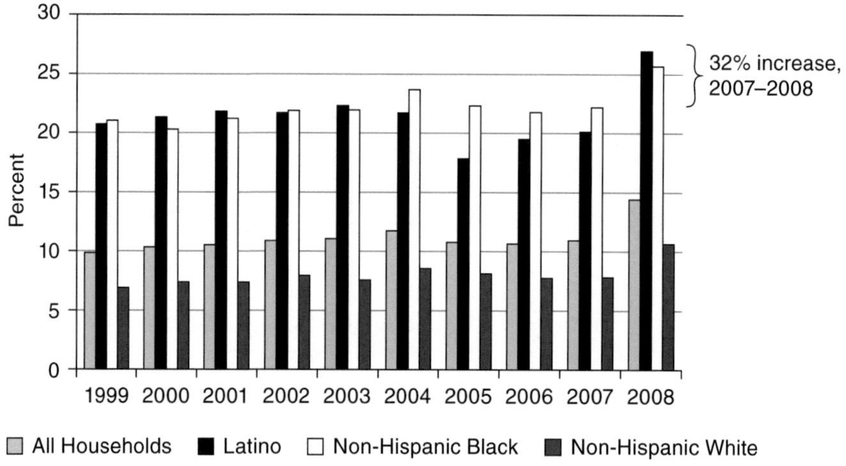

FIGURE 5-1 Proportion of food-insecure U.S. households (with and without children) by race and ethnic background, 1999–2008.
SOURCE: USDA/ERS (2000, 2002a, 2002b, 2003, 2004, 2005, 2006, 2007, 2008, 2009).

The Face of Food Security Over the Next Decades

Cook said that WIC will need to respond to changes in food insecurity over the next decades, but many questions remain regarding what those changes will be, such as:

- *Will poverty, food insecurity, and demand for food assistance remain persistently high or decrease?* Cook said that he views WIC as a food assistance program that was intended primarily to address the problem of food insecurity.
- *Will federal and state revenues continue to decline, remain where they are now, or increase?*
- *Will obesity-related health problems maintain pressure for food system reform and for further improvements in the WIC food packages?* Cook said that he views the use of WIC as a possible way to address the obesity epidemic.

Research Needed to Ensure WIC's Continued Effectiveness

Cook offered an extensive list of research topics, a number of which had been addressed in previous sessions:

1. How to reduce barriers to WIC participation;
2. How to assess the effectiveness and the true costs of functional ingredients added by manufacturers to approved WIC foods;
3. How to make more effective use of electronic benefit transfer (EBT) machines in WIC;
4. How WIC can more effectively encourage and support breastfeeding among participating mothers;
5. Ways to increase the use of WIC benefits in farmers markets, community-supported agriculture, and other venues that offer locally produced food;
6. Ways to increase funds available to WIC and to enable all eligible women, infants, and children to participate, with an emphasis on increasing participation by children;
7. Ways to further improve the quality of food purchased with WIC vouchers, especially in the smaller urban food stores that many WIC participants depend upon;
8. How to include oral health screening, fluoride treatment, dental sealant application, and other basic oral-health examination and referrals as part of WIC services, considering that poor oral health is a silent epidemic, especially in the pediatric population;

9. How to use WIC to help establish pediatric medical homes for infant and child participants; and
10. Additional, more rigorous evaluations of the effectiveness of WIC in
    a. Improving birth outcomes and reducing health care costs,
    b. Improving diet and diet-related outcomes for mothers and children,
    c. Improving infant feeding practices,
    d. Improving inter-natal and prenatal health and nutrition status, and
    e. Improving brain growth and cognitive development.

PERSPECTIVES ON WIC RESEARCH

Presenter: Edward A. Frongillo, Jr.[1]

When the National Nutrition Monitoring System was started, the view was that adverse effects of food insecurity occurred primarily as a function of poor dietary and nutritional status. Now, Frongillo said, it is known that many additional pathways affect well-being and health and help explain why food insecurity affects children's behavior, ability to learn, and many other aspects of their lives.

Prior Research on Food Insecurity and WIC

A paper by the U.S. Department of Agriculture Economic Research Service (USDA/ERS, 2009) found that approximately one-fourth of households that had received WIC benefits in the past 30 days had a food-insecure adult or child. Black et al. (2004) found a similar prevalence of food insecurity among those WIC participants and eligible non-participants who had access problems. Food insecurity has been associated with a poorer quality diet (Kropf et al., 2007). Bitler and Currie (2005) provided evidence that WIC reaches women and children who are at high nutritional risk. Herman and co-workers (2004) reported a reduction in food insecurity among postpartum women who had enrolled early in pregnancy. Furthermore, two-thirds of the women spent less money on food after enrolling in WIC; for one-third of the women, however, WIC benefits were used to complete the household food budget. Metallinos-Katsaras et al. (2010) also found that the risk of food insecurity with hunger was lower in the postpartum period for women who enrolled during the first or second trimester as opposed to the third trimester and, furthermore, that the risk of food insecurity for children decreased with each additional WIC visit by the mother.

[1]The literature review was conducted by Emily Heberlein.

Concepts of Food Insecurity

Food Insecurity as a Stressor

Three models address ways in which participation in WIC could modify the stressor effects of food insecurity: (1) WIC could eliminate the stressor, thereby improving outcomes; (2) WIC could compensate for the stress by providing assistance; or (3) WIC could serve as a buffer that interrupts the pathway between food insecurity and some outcomes. To illustrate his first model (the stress-elimination model), Frongillo discussed outcomes from an innovative program called BRAC's Ultra Poor program, which targeted the poorest 15 to 20 percent of the population in Bangladesh. The program decreased domestic violence dramatically, improved food security, improved the economic situation, and reduced social constraints. In this example, he said, a reduction in food insecurity accounted for about one-third of the substantial reduction in the distress (depression) of the participating women.

Frongillo also noted that early food supplementation of pregnant Bangladeshi women was accompanied by a higher mean birth weight and an improved quality of mother-infant interaction, but only among those with a high stress level (high food insecurity). By contrast, a peer-counseling lactation intervention provided more benefit to the women who were less stressed. A possible reason that only the women with lower stress levels benefited is that they were able to pay attention to messages and act on them, whereas the more highly stressed women were not.

Synergy Between Tangible Benefits and Behavior Changes

Just and Weninger (1997) provide evidence that the societal benefit from WIC and the Farmer's Market Nutrition Program arises when WIC coupons and information are given together. This work suggests that there may be a synergistic effect between the food voucher and behavior-change-communication components of WIC.

A model by Patterson (2002) suggests that an important question to answer is, "How can WIC help families achieve a balance between demands (stressors, strains, daily hassles) and their capabilities (resources, coping behaviors)?"

Research Questions

Frongillo offered the following list of research questions:

1. Does WIC reduce food insecurity, thereby leading to better outcomes?
2. Does WIC buffer the effects of food insecurity?
3. Does the food component of WIC primarily benefit those who are most food insecure?
4. Does the behavior-change-communication component of WIC primarily benefit those who are the *least* food insecure?
5. Does food insecurity need to be reduced by means of the WIC food package before communication to promote behavior change can be effective?
6. Does WIC reduce demands and increase capabilities, and how can WIC best help families balance these two coping strategies?

Closing Remarks

Frongillo closed his presentation by addressing points made in earlier presentations.

1. If WIC is connected with other programs and providers, the evidence from BRAC's Ultra Poor program suggests that a synergistic effect may occur. That is, the women's improved access to services and perceived higher social status in the community, combined with WIC benefits, may work together synergistically.
2. One possible outcome to monitor would be maternal–infant interactions, which can be measured on a fairly large scale, rather than birth weight, which Frongillo said is resistant to change.
3. Consideration needs to be given to possible gender differences when investigating outcomes among children.

RESPONSE

Discussant: James Weill

WIC's Purpose

Many people believe that the fundamental purpose of WIC is to reduce food insecurity that results from poverty, both because it should be unacceptable in our affluent society and because that strategy improves maternal and child health. Others believe WIC should be framed mainly as a public health program, in part because the severe hunger and malnutrition seen in the late 1960s and early 1970s are now uncommon. Weill said that this improvement is in large part due to the success of WIC and its sister nutrition assistance programs, but he asserted that this view of

WIC tends to underplay the connections between poverty, food insecurity, and poor health.

More people in the WIC age group are struggling financially than when WIC started. Comparing 1973 (essentially when WIC started) and 2007, median income adjusted for inflation decreased 23 percent, from $39,817 to $30,500, for households with children and headed by a person younger than 30 years of age. Moreover, 56 percent of these households had incomes below 200 percent of the poverty line in 2007 (prior to the great recession). Thus, in many ways, the economic struggle for young families has become worse since WIC began. Weill said that he considers WIC's role in addressing food insecurity to be just as important now as it was when WIC began.

Comments on Research Questions

Weill expressed agreement with research questions raised by Cook and Frongillo such as, "Does WIC reduce food insecurity?" and "For which populations does WIC buffer the effects of food insecurity?" Because the neediest subpopulation in WIC is probably the hardest to lift completely out of food insecurity, it is important to acknowledge that reaching that subpopulation is a desirable goal and to identify better ways to measure the positive effects of WIC, including moving families with *very low* food security up to low food security.

Weill said it is important to examine interactions of WIC with other programs, including the Supplemental Nutrition Assistance Program (SNAP) and Medicaid. Using SNAP as an example, he offered the following questions:

- Do WIC and SNAP together reduce food insecurity or very low food insecurity?; and, if so,
- Do they do it more robustly together than in isolation?
- Do the results differ for the different populations served by WIC?

The combination of WIC and Medicaid is especially important to address, given the phase-in of health care reform and the extension of Medicaid services to low-income women of childbearing age regardless of their parental or pregnancy status.

Other potential research topics include examining the effects of the food package on access to healthful foods in food deserts[2] and examining

[2]Food deserts are areas (typically rural or inner city areas) in which residents lack access to affordable healthful foods such as fruits, vegetables, whole grains, and low fat milk. Because vendors who participate in WIC must offer a selection of such foods, it would be possible for the food packages to improve access to healthful foods in food deserts.

whether WIC improves health and reduces obesity by improving food security. If it is true that improving food security can improve health and reduce obesity, it will be especially useful to examine ways to improve WIC's effect on food security.

GROUP DISCUSSION

Moderator: Maureen Black

Points made during the group discussion included the following:

- The effects of food insecurity may not be immediately visible in young children because those under 3 years of age may not experience effects on their weight or height.
- A two-item screen for households at risk for food insecurity was recently validated by Hager and colleagues (2010). One item addresses food, and the other addresses stress and anxiety in the household. The screening tool may be useful in pediatricians' offices and Social Security offices.
- The effects of food insecurity on childhood overweight appear to differ according to the maternal pre-pregnancy weight. Large sample sizes of low-income people will be needed to examine the influence of effect modifiers on the relationship between food insecurity and body weight.

SUMMARY OF SUGGESTED RESEARCH TOPICS

The research suggestions made during this session focused on ways to increase participation in WIC; to improve its effectiveness and the measurement of effectiveness; to examine relationships among WIC, food insecurity, and health outcomes; and to examine relationships among WIC, Medicaid, SNAP, food insecurity, and health outcomes. Studies may need to take into account the degree of food insecurity and how factors such as gender affect food insecurity.

REFERENCES

Anderson, S.A. 1990. Core indicators of nutritional state for difficult-to-sample populations. *Journal of Nutrition* 120:1557–1600.

Bitler, M. P., and J. Currie. 2005. Does WIC work? The effects of WIC on pregnancy and birth outcomes. *Journal of Policy Analysis and Management* 24(1):73–91.

Black, M. M., D. B. Cutts, D. A. Frank, J. Geppert, A. Skalicky, S. Levenson, P. H. Casey, C. Berkowitz, N. Zaldivar, J. T. Cook, A. F. Meyers, and T. Herren. 2004. Special Supplemental Nutrition Program for Women, Infants, and Children participation and infants' growth and health: A multisite surveillance study. *Pediatrics* 114(1):169–176.

Hager, E. R., A. M. Quigg, M. M. Black, S. M. Coleman, T. Heeren, R. Rose-Jacobs, J. T. Cook, S. A. de Cuba, P. H. Casey, M. Chilton, D. B. Cutts, A. F. Meyers, and D. A. Frank. 2010. Development and validity of a 2-item screen to identify families at risk for food insecurity. *Pediatrics* 126(1):e26–e32.

Herman, D. R., G. G. Harrison, A. A. Afifi, and E. Jenks. 2004. The effect of the WIC program on food security status of pregnant, first-time participants. *Family Economics & Nutrition Review* 16(1):21–29.

Just, R. E., and Q. Weninger. 1997. Economic evaluation of the Farmers' Market Nutrition Program. *American Journal of Agricultural Economics* 79:902–917.

Kropf, M. L., D. H. Holben, J. P. Holcomb, Jr., and H. Anderson. 2007. Food security status and produce intake and behaviors of Special Supplemental Nutrition Program for Women, Infants, and Children and farmers' market nutrition program participants. *Journal of the American Dietetic Association* 107(11):1903–1908.

Metallinos-Katsaras, E., K. S. Gorman, P. Wilde, and J. Kallio. 2010. A longitudinal study of WIC participation on household food insecurity. *Maternal and Child Health Journal.* http://www.springerlink.com/content/l12w4171117h5674/fulltext.pdf (published online May 9, 2010, accessed October 21, 2010)

Patterson, J. M. 2002. Understanding family resilience. *Journal of Clinical Psychology* 58: 233–246.

USDA/ERS (U.S. Department of Agriculture/Economic Research Service). 2000. *Household Food Security in the United States, 1999.* Washington, DC: USDA/ERS. http://www.ers.usda.gov/publications/fanrr8/fanrr8.pdf (accessed September 17, 2010).

USDA/ERS. 2002a. *Household Food Security in the United States, 2000.* Washington, DC: USDA/ERS. http://www.ers.usda.gov/publications/fanrr21/fanrr21.pdf (accessed September 17, 2010).

USDA/ERS. 2002b. *Household Food Security in the United States, 2001.* Washington, DC: USDA/ERS. http://www.ers.usda.gov/publications/fanrr29/fanrr29.pdf (accessed September 17, 2010).

USDA/ERS. 2003. *Household Food Security in the United States, 2002.* Washington, DC: USDA/ERS. http://www.ers.usda.gov/publications/fanrr35/fanrr35.pdf (accessed September 17, 2010).

USDA/ERS. 2004. *Household Food Security in the United States, 2003.* Washington, DC: USDA/ERS. http://www.ers.usda.gov/publications/fanrr42/fanrr42.pdf (accessed September 17, 2010).

USDA/ERS. 2005. *Household Food Security in the United States, 2004.* Washington, DC: USDA/ERS. http://www.ers.usda.gov/publications/err11/err11.pdf (accessed September 17, 2010).

USDA/ERS. 2006. *Household Food Security in the United States, 2005.* Washington, DC: USDA/ERS. http://www.ers.usda.gov/Publications/ERR29/ERR29.pdf (accessed September 17, 2010).

USDA/ERS. 2007. *Household Food Security in the United States, 2006.* Washington, DC: USDA/ERS. http://www.ers.usda.gov/Publications/ERR29/ERR29.pdf (accessed September 17, 2010).

USDA/ERS. 2008. *Household Food Security in the United States, 2007.* Washington, DC: USDA/ERS. http://www.ers.usda.gov/Publications/ERR66/ERR66.pdf (accessed September 17, 2010).

USDA/ERS. 2009. *Household Food Security in the United States, 2008.* Washington, DC: USDA/ERS. http://www.ers.usda.gov/publications/err83/err83.pdf (accessed September 15, 2010).

6

Dietary Intake and Nutritional Status

Barbara Devaney, the session's moderator, began the session by pointing out that, of the three major components of the Special Supplemental Nutrition Program for Women, Infants, and Children (WIC), the WIC food packages account for the largest proportion of WIC dollars spent. Moreover, the food packages are rich sources of the foods and nutrients known to be lacking in the diets of low-income women, infants, and children. Thus, a key question is how effective WIC is in changing the dietary intakes of its participants.

This session focused on the research agenda for studying the effects of WIC on dietary intakes. Nancy Cole addressed potential research concerning the dietary intake and nutritional status of women and children, and Nancy Krebs addressed research related to infants. Discussant Suzanne Murphy responded by focusing on an approach to address the research questions.

WOMEN AND CHILDREN

Presenter: Nancy Cole

WIC provides a package of foods for women and children with the objective of promoting healthful food choices, improving dietary intake, and improving nutritional status. Cole's presentation considered which elements to examine when conducting research on the impact of the WIC food package and included suggestions for research related to each of these.

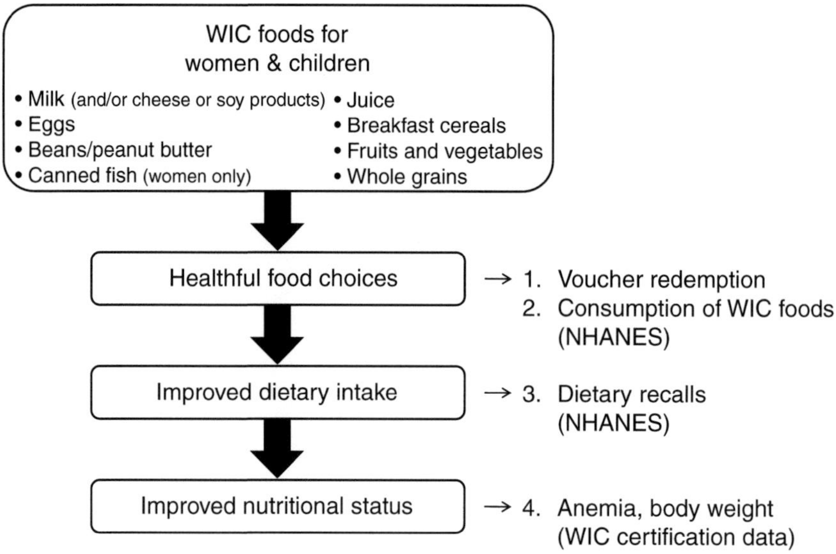

FIGURE 6-1 Measures for studying the impact of WIC food packages on women and children. NOTE: NHANES = National Health and Nutrition Examination Survey. SOURCE: Cole (2010).

Figure 6-1 illustrates measures that might be used for studying the impact of WIC food packages.

Early Steps Involving the WIC Food Package

To address the question of whether WIC improves dietary intakes and nutritional status, it is useful to consider two early steps as they relate to the food package: voucher pick-up and redemption, and the consumption of WIC foods.

Voucher Redemption

Prior research Administrative data are available that can be used to examine voucher pick-up and redemption, but they have seldom been used. The WIC Cost Containment Study (USDA/ERS, 2003) found that voucher pick-up across six states declined during the certification period, dropping from about 100 percent in the first month to between 73 and 84 percent by the sixth month.

Potential research Potential research on voucher redemption could include the following topics:

1. The impact of the revised WIC food packages on redemption, using a pre-versus-post comparison study or looking across states to observe the effects of differences in state policies (e.g., those specifying allowed foods), and
2. The effect of the revised WIC food packages on changes in redemption rates during the certification period and features of the revised packages to which the changes could be attributed.

Consumption of WIC Foods

Prior research Relatively little information is available concerning the extent to which WIC foods are consumed by WIC participants. Dietary data from the National Health and Nutrition Examination surveys (NHANES) during the period 1999–2004 have been used for this purpose. For example, the Food and Nutrition Service of the U.S. Department of Agriculture (USDA) reported that children participating in WIC were significantly more likely than other low-income children to consume WIC-approved cereals (USDA/FNS, 2008). However, NHANES data have a number of weaknesses: They cannot be used to measure impact, sample sizes are small for the populations of interest, and state identifiers are lacking. Cole stated that much can be learned from asking participants why they consumed only some or none of the WIC foods.

Potential research Potential research could examine the marginal effect of various factors on WIC participants' consumption of WIC foods by determining the following:

1. The percentages of the foods in the food package consumed by the participant and by other family members, and
2. Variation of the WIC food consumption rate by category of food in the revised food packages—specifically, new foods, food categories with increased substitution, and food categories with decreased quantities.

Dietary Intake

Prior research on dietary intake has largely involved descriptive studies based on NHANES data. The studies have indicated that nearly all children from 1 through 4 years of age had adequate usual daily intake of all the vitamins (except E) and minerals that have defined Estimated Average Requirements.

Potential research to address the effect of revised WIC food packages on dietary intake could use the following approaches:

1. Replicate an earlier NHANES analysis in the period after implementation of the revised food packages; and
2. Use the Centers for Disease Control and Prevention Research Data Center to control for characteristics of state WIC food lists, which differ in the amount of choice allowed within each food category. Cole suggested that participating children in states with restrictive WIC food lists would provide a valid control group for lower-bound estimates of the impact of WIC; however, sample sizes in those states may be relatively small.

Nutritional and Health Status

The WIC Cost Containment Study (USDA/ERS, 2003) used a dose-response approach to estimating WIC impacts on nutritional status and health, with voucher redemption as the dose measurement. Using this method, WIC was found to have statistically significant beneficial effects on change in height for age and on probabilities related to the risk of underweight and anemia.

The following two possible descriptive analyses of change in nutritional and health status make use of the WIC Participants and Program Characteristics (WIC-PC) data:

1. For a sample of states, obtain a second WIC-PC extract 6 months after the WIC-PC submission and examine changes in status; and
2. Follow the approach in (1) but also obtain measures of voucher redemption for use in a dose-response analysis.

Summary of Potential Research

In summary, Cole's research suggestions covered four topics related to the food package and dietary intake:

- *Voucher redemption* Trends before and after revised food packages
- *Consumption of WIC foods* (1) Analysis of NHANES and comparison of recent WIC food consumption with consumption before the implementation of revised food packages, possibly controlling for characteristics of states' food lists; and (2) a new survey to understand the marginal effect of WIC on the consumption of WIC foods and reasons for not consuming the full WIC food package
- *Dietary intakes* NHANES analysis of usual daily intakes of nutrients by WIC participants and non-participants compared with intakes before implementation of revised food packages

- *Nutritional/health status* Analysis of administrative data from a sample of states

INFANTS AND YOUNG CHILDREN

Presenter: Nancy Krebs

In her presentation, Krebs reviewed data relating to dietary intake, growth, and iron status and provided the rationale for her WIC research priorities.

Dietary Intake

Data from the first Feeding Infant and Toddlers Study (FITS) (Ponza et al., 2004) indicate that at least 95 percent of infants 4 through 11 months of age consumed infant formula. Although 95 percent of the infants ages 7 through 11 months of age consumed cereals and purees, fewer than 5 percent consumed meats (the best sources of iron and zinc), and more than 50 percent consumed sweets and desserts.

FITS data indicate that less than 1 percent of formula-fed infants had usual nutrient intakes that were lower than the Estimated Average Requirement or mean intakes that were lower than the Adequate Intake. However, substantial proportions of breastfed infants had inadequate intakes of iron or zinc or both. Many infants in FITS were reported to have excessive energy intakes (Ponza et al., 2004).

In a study of children's diet quality using the Healthy Eating Index as a standard, the Food and Nutrition Service compared the diets of WIC participants and eligible non-participants (USDA/FNS, 2008). Although the diets of the two groups were generally comparable, none were consistent with the *Dietary Guidelines for Americans*. The investigators suggested that measures be taken to reduce children's intake of saturated fat and sweetened beverages and to increase their intakes of whole grains, whole fruit (as opposed to juice), and a variety of vegetables (rather than mainly potatoes). The revised WIC food packages are well aligned with these suggested dietary changes.

Growth

In her analysis, Krebs used data on infant growth from a study by Black et al. (2004) that compared infants on WIC with those not on WIC because of access problems. In particular, Krebs converted *z* scores for length and weight to approximate percentiles, and she found that the means for both groups were well within the normal range on the Centers for Disease Control and Prevention (CDC) growth chart. She concluded that although the differences observed, including the modest shift of the overall distributions of growth parameters, were statistically significant, they were unlikely to be clinically important.

The World Health Organization (WHO) growth charts for breastfed infants (de Onis, 2006; WHO, 2010) differ from the 2000 CDC growth charts for infants (CDC, 2010a; Kuczmarski et al., 2000). Krebs illustrated this by plotting the 3rd, 50th, and 97th CDC percentiles on a WHO chart (Figure 6-2), and she noted that this difference has implications for evaluating growth.

Iron Status

Analyses of NHANES data have shown a marked decrease in the prevalence of iron deficiency anemia among infants and young children since 1971, but Krebs pointed out that this is very likely the result of encouraging the feeding of iron-fortified formula and the decrease in the use of whole cow milk (Cusik et al., 2008). (Krebs noted that the intake of iron-fortified cereal has been reported to decrease by infants' eighth month.) Reported rates of iron deficiency in toddlers from the NHANES data range from 6.6 percent to 15.2 percent; for iron deficiency anemia they range from 0.9 to 4.4 percent. Higher rates have been reported in smaller series that include high-risk subpopulations.

Proposed Research Priorities

Priority One

According to Krebs, the highest priority for WIC research should be how to increase breastfeeding rates in the United States. Addressing this question would require a change in the culture and administration of WIC to allow interventional research.

Rationale In Krebs' opinion, the data are overwhelmingly conclusive that WIC undermines breastfeeding in the United States. She said that the positive effects of breastfeeding-promotion programs, peer counseling, and related efforts are dwarfed by the provision of free formula for a full year. This free-formula policy is unique to the United States and is contrary to the Baby Friendly Hospital Initiative, the International Code of Marketing, and the global efforts of WHO to promote breastfeeding. A lack of breastfeeding has profound adverse health effects for infants, women, and society.

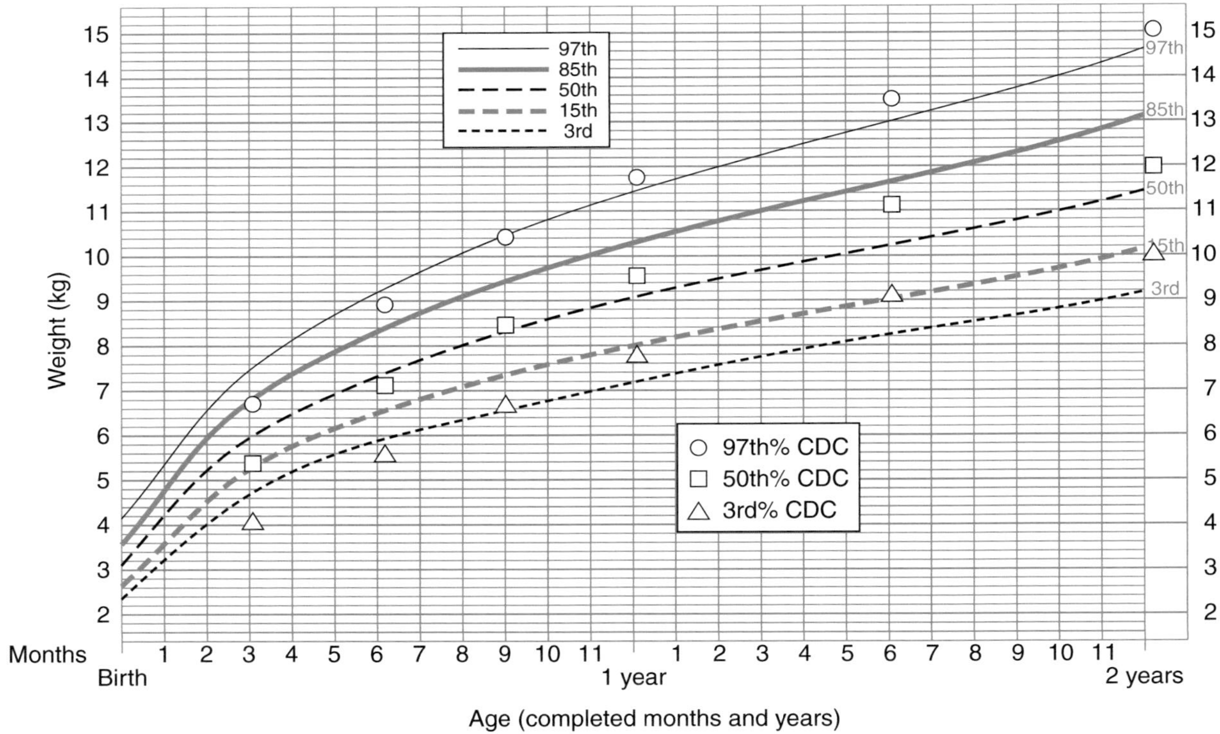

FIGURE 6-2 A comparison of CDC and WHO weight-for-age percentiles from birth to 2 years for girls. The WHO charts covering birth to 2 years were developed using data on breastfed children (de Onis et al., 2006). CDC now recommends that WHO growth standards be used in the United States for this age group (CDC, 2010b).
NOTE: CDC = Centers for Disease Control and Prevention, WHO = World Health Organization.
SOURCES: CDC (2010a); WHO (2010). Reprinted with permission from WHO.

Proposed study design Krebs' proposal was to use a cluster-randomized trial to test the effect of not providing free formula for any infant from birth to 6 months of age (which is not the same as formula not being used at all). She suggested measuring the following outcomes: rates and duration of breastfeeding, growth and nutritional status from 0 to 24 months of age, dietary quality and feeding practices from 0 to 24 months of age, maternal body mass index at 6 months, medical expenses and utilization, and WIC participation rates.

Other Research Priorities

Because of time constraints, Krebs did not discuss her other research priorities, but she did quickly show slides that covered them. They are summarized in Box 6-1.

Summary

In closing, Krebs again emphasized that the nutritional status of infants and toddlers who are WIC participants is currently dominated by the use of formula. If and when breastfeeding rates increase, the entire care team will need to be aware of the importance of complementary feeding and of how to prevent and treat deficiencies. The beneficial impact of increasing breastfeeding duration could be profound.

BOX 6-1
Other Research Priorities

- *Priority 2* Evaluate the impact of WIC participation on growth outcomes using the World Health Organization growth standards (0–24 months), determining outcomes such as the percentages of overweight and underweight infants and effects of the early rate of weight gain on later weight outcomes.
- *Priority 3* Evaluate the impact of new WIC food packages with regard to breastfeeding rates and duration, formula use by partially breastfed infants, and formula feeding, measuring outcomes such as feeding practices, growth, iron status, and health status and medical expenditures for both the infant and the mother.
- *Priority 4* Evaluate the impact of the new infant and child food packages on diet quality and nutritional status, examining the association of meat intake at 6 months with iron status in breastfed infants and both immediate and longer-term effects of the revised food package.

RESPONSE

Discussant: Suzanne Murphy

Murphy pointed out that the report *WIC Food Packages: Time for a Change* (IOM, 2006), for which she served as chairperson, includes a chapter on recommendations about evaluations of the revised WIC food package and identifies a number of variables to examine in such evaluations. In addition, Murphy described the importance of conducting periodic national evaluations of WIC. NHANES has strong clinical measures, but it is cross-sectional and has very limited samples of pregnant and lactating women and breastfed infants. A WIC survey, on the other hand, could track attitudes and behaviors, food purchasing patterns, the use of vouchers, and the mother-child dyad. It also could allow comparisons among the larger states. A longitudinal study could track changes in the health of the same WIC women and children over time and compare them with a control group. Other advantages of a periodic WIC survey, Murphy said, would be increased visibility of the program to the public and to Congress and the development of a source of data that might provide justification for funding WIC at a relatively high level.

Murphy suggested that outcomes could be tracked over time with NHANES and NHANES follow-ups if modules were added to those surveys that included additional details on WIC usage. A national WIC survey with a longitudinal component would be an attractive alternative to determine whether WIC has a long-term effect on the health of children that participate in the program. The goal would be to complement other types of research, not to replace them. Funding for a WIC survey might be sought from Congress. A recurring survey would provide justification for a consistent level of funding to support this activity.

GROUP DISCUSSION

Moderator: Barbara Devaney

Much of the discussion centered on Krebs' suggested study that would examine the effects of providing no free formula to WIC mothers for the first 6 months after giving birth. Hirschman said that USDA does not have the authority to conduct the type of study proposed; an act of Congress would be required. Many of the comments included strong support for breastfeeding but raised concerns about Krebs' proposal. The suggested alternate approaches included:

- Allow free formula, but make it more difficult to obtain.
- Consider providing only generically labeled formula.
- Engage all care providers in support for breastfeeding.
- Time breastfeeding messages appropriately.
- Intensify support for all mothers in providing early infant feeding that is adequate and appropriate.
- Establish an environment in the United States in which breastfeeding is not viewed as painful, too much work, or insufficient for the infant and in which women can continue breastfeeding even if working.

SUMMARY OF SUGGESTED RESEARCH TOPICS

The first set of research proposals made during the session focused on ways to examine the dietary and nutrient intake of women and children, including analyzing data on voucher redemption and the consumption of WIC foods. Careful analyses of state administrative data would provide useful information. The second major proposal was for a cluster-randomized controlled trial to examine how to increase breastfeeding in the United States. The third major proposal was for a longitudinal study, perhaps as a part of a periodic national WIC survey, to track a variety of outcomes associated with WIC participation.

REFERENCES

Black, M. M., D. B. Cutts, D. A. Frank, J. Geppert, A. Skalicky, S. Levenson, P. H. Casey, C. Berkowitz, N. Zaldivar, J. T. Cook, A. F. Meyers, and T. Herren. 2004. Special Supplemental Nutrition Program for Women, Infants, and Children participation and infants' growth and health: A multisite surveillance study. *Pediatrics* 114(1):169–176.

CDC (Centers for Disease Control and Prevention). 2010a. *CDC Growth Charts*. http://www.cdc.gov/growthcharts/cdc_charts.htm (accessed September 24, 2010).

CDC. 2010b. *WHO Growth Standards Are Recommended for Use in the U.S. for Infants and Children 0 to 2 Years of Age*. http://www.cdc.gov/growthcharts/who_charts.htm (accessed September 24, 2010).

Cole, N. 2010. *Dietary intake and nutritional status: Women and children*. Presented at the Institute of Medicine Workshop on Health Impacts of WIC—Planning a Research Agenda, Washington, DC, July 20–21.

Cusick, S. E., Z. Mei, D. S. Freedman, A. C. Looker, C. L. Ogden, E. Gunter, and M. E. Cogswell. 2008. Unexplained decline in the prevalence of anemia among us children and women between 1988–1994 and 1999–2002. *American Journal of Clinical Nutrition* 88(6):1611–1617.

de Onis, M. 2006. WHO Child Growth Standards based on length/height, weight and age. *Acta Paediatrica, International Journal of Paediatrics* 95(Suppl. 450):76–85.

IOM (Institute of Medicine). 2006. *WIC Food Packages: Time for a Change*. Washington, DC: The National Academies Press.

Kuczmarski, R. J., C. L. Ogden, L. M. Grummer-Strawn, K. M. Flegal, S. S. Guo, R. Wei, Z. Mei, L. R. Curtin, A. F. Roche, and C. L. Johnson. 2000. CDC growth charts: United States. *Advance Data from Vital and Health Statistics* (314):1–27. http://www.cdc.gov/nchs/data/ad/ad314.pdf (accessed September 24, 2010).

Ponza, M., B. Devaney, P. Ziegler, K. Reidy, and C. Squatrito. 2004. Nutrient intakes and food choices of infants and toddlers participating in WIC. *Journal of the American Dietetic Association* 104(Suppl. 1):S71–S79.

USDA/ERS (U.S. Department of Agriculture/Economic Research Service). 2003. *Assessment of WIC Cost-Containment Practices: Final Report.* Washington, DC: USDA/ERS. http://www.ers.usda.gov/publications/efan03005/efan03005.pdf (accessed September 2, 2010).

USDA/FNS (U.S. Department of Agriculture/Food and Nutrition Service). 2008. *Diet Quality of American Young Children by WIC Participation Status: Data from the National Health and Nutrition Examination Survey, 1999–2004.* Alexandria, VA: USDA/FNS. http://www.fns.usda.gov/ora/menu/Published/WIC/FILES/NHANES-WIC.pdf (accessed September 2, 2010).

WHO (World Health Organization). 2010. *The WHO child growth standards.* http://www.who.int/childgrowth/standards/en (accessed September 24, 2010).

7

Nutrition Education in WIC

The two presentations in this session, moderated by Shannon Whaley, represent a collaborative effort of the two presenters, Lorrene Ritchie and Marilyn Townsend. Ritchie presented an overview of past studies; then Townsend addressed research design and timing and introduced a joint proposal for a study. The discussants (Maureen Black and Loren Bell) expanded on the presentations and raised additional questions. All five participants in this session are members of the nutrition education group mentioned later in this chapter.

OVERVIEW OF PAST STUDIES

Presenter: Lorrene Ritchie

Nutrition education in the Special Supplemental Nutrition Program for Women, Infants, and Children (WIC) involves helping participants understand the importance of nutrition and physical activity to their health and also learn how to make positive changes in those habits with the goal of reducing health risks including obesity. The process of delivering nutrition education in WIC is illustrated in Figure 7-1. The boxes in the figure each contain several entries because effective nutrition education interventions may involve components from several teaching approaches and delivery mediums. The review of studies that follows was intended to illustrate specific points and characterize the current state of knowledge on nutrition education in WIC.

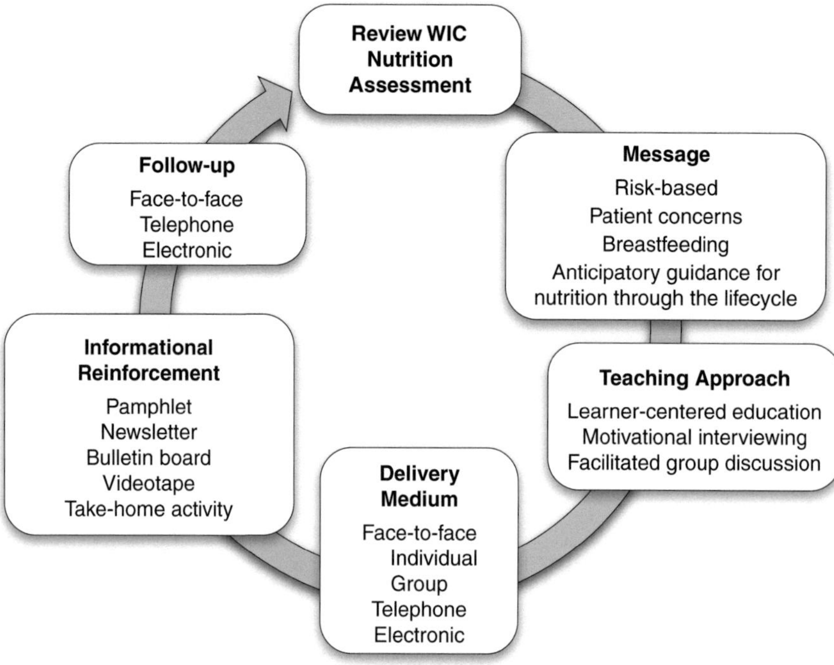

FIGURE 7-1 Process of delivering nutrition education in WIC.
SOURCE: USDA/National Agricultural Library (2006).

Participant Needs

The first rule in most behavior change models is to adapt the approach so as to best meet the participants' needs. Studies on participant needs have shown that 80 to 95 percent of WIC participants indicated satisfaction with the nutrition education (Nestor et al., 2001; USDA/FNS, 2000), but they also identified barriers, such as repetition and a lack of activities available for the children while they were waiting for their mothers (Woelfel et al., 2004). Participant preferences included child care, facilitated discussions, more talking by the participants, and cooking classes.

Approaches

Most of the studies on approaches have been of the type called *WIC plus studies*, in which augmented WIC services are compared with the usual services using convenience samples. Findings from these studies can be used to inform efforts to improve the delivery of WIC nutrition education, but these studies are not necessarily representative of usual practice or the resources normally available in WIC. Facilitated group discussion has been shown to improve self-efficacy (Abusabha et al., 1998) but not knowledge (USDA/FNS, 2001a) or maternal weight (Krummel et al., 2010). In other studies, learner-centered education improved folate intake (Cena et al., 2008) and the adoption of practices consistent with increasing fruit and vegetable intake (Gerstein et al., 2010). Havas et al. (1998) reported that peer education and support improved knowledge, led to a higher stage of change,[1] increased self-efficacy, and increased the intake of fruits and vegetables. Similarly, Ikeda and colleagues (2002) reported that peer support increased the intake of several important food groups. On the other hand, Chang et al. (2010) reported no effect of peer education on diet or body weight. Whaley and colleagues (2010) reported that motivational interviewing had beneficial effects on children's dietary and TV habits. Ritchie noted that she had found no studies that compared individual one-on-one education to group education approaches.

Messages

Ritchie identified studies that address four of the many subjects that are part of the WIC educational effort: cooking (Birmingham et al., 2004; Tessaro et al., 2007), low-fat milk (Ritchie et al., 2010; USDA/ERS, 2007), physical activity (Fahrenwald et al., 2004), and fruit and vegetable education plus coupons (Anderson et al., 2001; Whaley, submitted). In most cases, the studies found significant effects on behavior change and attitudes. Few studies have used randomized controlled designs, however. The question remains, "What messages are most important to address with WIC participants?"

Audience

Most of the WIC nutrition education studies address pregnant or postpartum women (USDA/FNS, 2000). Few have been targeted at preschool children (USDA/FNS, 2001b) or staff (Crawford et al., 2004).

Technology

The use of technology is emerging as a way to provide nutrition education to a larger number of WIC participants, with the additional goal of doing it in a cost-effective manner. Relatively few studies have been published on the use of new technological methods. The ones Ritchie reviewed examined a website (Bensley et al., 2006), touch screen video (USDA/FNS,

[1]For information about the Stages of Change model, see Prochaska et al. (1992).

2001a), interactive CD-ROMs (Block et al., 2000; Campbell et al., 2004), and computer kiosks (Carroll et al., 1996; Trepka et al., 2010). The studies suggest that technological methods are well-liked, but their impact and cost-effectiveness are not well known.

State-Wide Campaigns

Three state-wide nutrition education campaigns have reported positive results in modifying participant behaviors, but the results depended on using the participants as their own controls and examining their behavior pre- and post-campaign. Furthermore, the studies were limited by not including comparisons to other approaches to delivering nutrition education in WIC. The topics of the campaigns included television viewing (Johnson et al., 2005), family meals (Johnson et al., 2006), and new foods in the WIC food packages (Ritchie et al., 2010).

FUTURE RESEARCH

Presenter: Marilyn Townsend

Research Design and Timing

After reviewing studies of WIC nutrition education, Townsend said that the most common design had used a pretest followed by an intervention and then a posttest. It would be valuable to consider more complex designs, she said. To improve study designs, more attention should be paid to the possibility of longitudinal design, random selection and assignment to minimize selection bias, appropriate comparison or control groups, multivariate analysis to account for moderating variables, validated outcome measures, the use of a number of states and sites to take the research beyond the clinic level of delivery and analysis, and the method of data collection.

Suggested Reporting Methods

Adoption of TREND statement for describing study To achieve more systematic reviews of WIC interventions and possibly to allow for the merging of small datasets, Townsend and Ritchie recommended that investigators follow the Transparent Reporting of Evaluations with Nonrandomized Designs (TREND) statement (Des Jarlias et al., 2004) when reporting primary prevention intervention (nutrition education) studies related to WIC, whether non-randomized or randomized. Developed by 26 journal editors and experts from the Centers for Disease Control and Prevention, the TREND statement identifies 22 critical elements that should be included in reports. In particular, researchers should be careful to provide detailed information on intervention timing, dosage, effect size, intervention content, control content, participant assignment, and the unit of analysis.

Strategy statement for describing intervention A strategy statement is a description of the procedures used in the intervention that is detailed enough that another investigator could replicate the intervention. Such a strategy statement involves the systematic specification of each theory-driven strategy used in the intervention. Such information is crucial, Townsend emphasized, because we do not yet know what behavioral change strategies work with WIC clients, and we need to uncover what works, how well each strategy works, and why it works. Michie and Abraham (2004) investigated behavior change interventions in many health education fields and identified 26 evidence-based techniques or strategies, five of which appeared to be especially important (Michie et al., 2009).

Potential Research Questions

Townsend identified eight categories pertaining to research on nutrition education in WIC: the subject of the research, dose, approach, delivery, reinforcement and follow-up, educators, participants, and data sets.

Subject Townsend suggested that the following questions be considered: Should the focus be on obesity prevention? Should the research be organized as campaigns with common themes and timelines? Should it include child feeding and development or cooking and shopping, or both?

Dose Information is needed on whether four education contacts per year are sufficient, how session attendance can be increased, and whether WIC nutrition education contacts are synergistic with other nutrition education programs, such as Head Start and Supplemental Nutrition Assistance Program-Education (SNAP-Ed).

Approach There are insufficient data regarding the optimal approaches to WIC nutrition education, including the cost-effectiveness of the various approaches. These approaches include learner-centered education, facilitated group discussion, peer-led discussions, motivational negotiation, anticipatory guidance, and interactive or experiential education (such as cooking demonstrations, taste testing, field trips).

Delivery Similarly, there are insufficient data about the optimal methods of delivery. In addition to the methods mentioned by Ritchie, methods to consider might include home or workplace visits and contacts in the WIC waiting area.

Reinforcement and follow-up Among the reinforcing approaches that could be tested are email or text messages, take-home materials, social marketing, self-monitoring (see Havas et al., 1998, for an example), and other home activities.

Educators Key questions concerning the educators or "messengers" might include the following: To what extent is staff wellness important? What are the components of optimal training and staff development for nutrition educators? What are the best methods to reduce turnover?

Participants It is unclear to what extent nutrition education should be directed at children or significant others, or both; and little is known about overcoming the barriers to effective nutrition education.

Data sets The nutrition education group agreed that no existing data sets would provide the information needed to address the questions that need to be studied.

Proposed Study

As a next step in research design, Townsend and Ritchie proposed a study that would be less expensive than a national study. The study addresses the question, "Can WIC nutrition education reduce the risk of obesity?" The proposed elements of the study are:

- *Delivery approaches* Within the WIC population, compare the impacts of three delivery approaches: (1) a learner-centered model (a group at a clinic), (2) an online learning-at-home model (an individual at home), and (3) a counseling model as a control (one-on-one at clinic).
- *Design* In each of four to six states with different demographics, select eight clinics: four for approach 1, and four for approach 3 (above). The online clients (approach 2) should be volunteers recruited from all the study clinics.

Because of a lack of appropriate controls, Townsend said the study would need to focus on relative differences. Results from different sites could be merged using appropriate analyses. The proposed design would be an informative next step and would be less expensive than a national study.

RESPONSE

Discussant: Maureen Black

After showing video clips that illustrated some mother–child interactions, Black briefly addressed aspects of mealtime and food behaviors; policy, environmental, and developmental issues that could influence or be a part of nutrition education in WIC; and methodological issues related to education and behavior change.

Mealtime and Food Behaviors

Maternal feeding behaviors are influenced by the infant or child's behavior, as can be clearly seen by observing a mother–infant dyad when breastfeeding. Children's intake is influenced by the availability of food; the mealtime context; and mealtime interactions with the caregiver, which might be responsive, controlling, indulgent, or uninvolved. Several studies report negative effects of excessive control (Faith et al., 2004; Fisher and Birch, 1999, 2002; Lee et al., 2001). The reasons that parents may exert excessive control include concerns about the child's health and body size, time constraints, and food insecurity. Building on concepts from the field of child development, investigators have begun to study whether responsive feeding leads to healthful mealtime behavior and then to healthful growth.

Other Topics Pertinent to Nutrition Education

Black noted that the following topics, which had been mentioned earlier in the workshop, are relevant to nutrition education: topics in the areas of policies and economics, family structure and function, prenatal development, and obesity. She then added two relevant topics to the list: the "nutrition transition," which is characterized by an easy access to ready-to-eat food and reduced energy expenditure; and infants' and toddlers' increasing desire for autonomy.

Methodological Issues and Strategies

Because didactic education has limitations, WIC has incorporated learner-centered education, tailored messages, and various other strategies, such as motivational interviewing to elicit change. Knowledge and intentions are necessary but not sufficient for effecting behavioral change. Black reminded the audience that research questions related to dose and incentives were raised by previous presenters.

BOX 7-1
Comparative Effectiveness Design Elements

1. Measure target outcome
2. Assign persons to an educational strategy (e.g., individual or group), possibly by random
3. Deliver education
4. Measure target outcome and client satisfaction
5. Compare outcomes across differing educational strategies

Black proposed that research take the form of comparative effectiveness studies. With this method, intervention A is compared with intervention B rather than with a control group. The basic elements in this method are given in Box 7-1. With replication and the sharing of findings across sites, this strategy could lead to quality improvement within WIC and to more integrated systems.

RESPONSE

Discussant: Loren Bell

Bell began his response by providing context for his perspectives and then suggested a number of topics for research.

Context

Bell's food assistance and nutrition research team has a project covering a number of states, most of which are in the U.S. Department of Agriculture's (USDA's) western region but some of which are in the mountain plains and the Midwest. Over approximately the past 4 years, team members have visited 19 states and 60 local WIC agencies. They have conducted Web surveys, interviewed more than 600 local WIC staff who provide nutrition education, held focus groups or intercept interviews with 1,800 WIC clients about nutrition education, and observed the delivery of services.

The team members observed very large variations in the delivery of nutrition education and identified three major issues. The first issue concerned the demands of the WIC computer system and the need to document eligibility. The staff may be unable to apply their skills in learner-centered approaches, for example, because of the need to ask many specific computer-directed questions, many of which the client may not understand. The second issue is the widespread use of a deficit model. In response to this issue, the research team has been focusing on the affirmation of positive behaviors as a potentially more effective approach to behavior change. The third issue is effective use of time. Staff members indicate that they have insufficient time for learner-centered education; whereas the clients have long waiting times.

Suggested Topics for Research

A major emphasis of the project that Bell's team has been carrying out is the design of evaluation methodologies to determine outcomes that are reasonable given what can actually be accomplished in the WIC site. Based on findings from that project, Bell identified seven major questions for research:

1. *How is nutrition education delivered?* The context should be framed before the interventions are described.
2. *How can one evaluate the intervention in view of interventions from other programs?* Because it is nearly impossible to separate the effects of a WIC intervention from a SNAP-Ed nutrition intervention[2] (assuming that both are directed toward promoting the same behavior change, such as the consumption of low-fat milk), it is important to be realistic and practical concerning what can be measured in WIC.
3. *What kind of outcome is desired?* Questions arise about the significance of moving to a higher stage of change (for example, moving from the contemplation stage to the preparation stage, when one actually prepares to make a specific change) and of making specific behavioral changes.
4. *How do clients like to learn?* Focus groups and intervention intercept interviews have indicated that clients are open to the use of electronic media, both for nutrition education contacts and reminders or messages.
5. *How do factors that contribute to health disparities relate to nutrition education?* How far a mother lives from a grocery store that carries fresh fruits and vegetables is an example of a factor that should be considered in nutrition education.
6. *What is WIC's role in providing nutrition education services to postpartum women and significant others?* Women reported feeling

---

[2]SNAP-Ed nutrition interventions refer to nutrition education efforts directed to persons eligible for SNAP, not to the provision of monthly benefits that can be used for the purchase of foods.

ignored because the attention is focused on the baby or on breastfeeding. Males said that WIC has nothing to offer them.

7. *How should self-reporting by clients be addressed?* Members of focus groups reported that the best thing about WIC is the people. One reason given for erroneous self-reporting was that WIC participants did not want to disappoint staff.

Closing Remarks

Although many issues concerning nutrition education will need to be addressed in the future, Bell urged the initial focus to be on what nutrition education is and then on the appropriate outcome for the interventions.

GROUP DISCUSSION

Moderator: Shannon E. Whaley

The wide-ranging discussion involved many participants and addressed a number of points, which are summarized below:

- *Methods for reaching out to clients* WIC health professionals and clients appear to have different views about the preferred methods for reaching out to clients. One survey of WIC personnel listed fact sheets, brochures and pamphlets, and recipes, while the clients said they would like WIC to use text messages and social networking. Even clients in the Pacific Islands are using electronic media and would like WIC to do so also. It was noted that preferences are often expressed in terms of an idealized state rather than with consideration to what will actually work well. In California, for example, a decline in literacy has been noted among low-income clientele, raising questions about how to reach them effectively. Not enough research has been conducted to determine the extent to which electronic media can be used in WIC and whether it will have any effect on nutrition.
- *Social networking* There is considerable evidence that social networks have power to influence behavior change. The theory behind social learning is well-established, involving such basic concepts as modeling and outcome expectancies. Small electronic social networks might be created that could operate and have influence beyond the site of the intervention.
- *Partnerships with other programs* To move the research agenda forward, it could be useful to work together with other programs (e.g., SNAP-Ed) and share the burden of research.

- *Reporting of research findings in journals* The TREND guidance for reporting research findings is valuable. The extent to which investigators are following the guidance is not being evaluated (however, the development of rating scales was suggested for this purpose), and many journal editors are publishing papers that do not conform to the guidance statement. Because researchers cannot stay within the maximum word count for articles if they provide all the information specified in the guidance, alternative ways to provide the information (such as an addendum to an electronic version of the article) need to be found.
- *Evaluation of individual WIC programs* Questions arose regarding the methods that USDA uses to evaluate individual programs, specifically related to the fact that the monitoring methods tend to focus on the negative. Some states have restructured their monitoring tools to emphasize an approach based on positive affirmation rather than addressing only what was wrong.
- *Maternal factors* Nutrition education needs to consider maternal depression, different temperaments, and general parenting skills. It was noted that some caregivers do not recognize that they are using food for a behavioral purpose (e.g., giving food to a child to calm the child).
- *Humor* Consider ways to make learning fun.

SUMMARY OF SUGGESTED RESEARCH TOPICS

The research suggestions made during this session focused on methods and on nutrition education strategies that are intended to reduce the risk of obesity. Many research questions were raised concerning identification of the message, message delivery, appropriate outcomes, consideration of environmental effects and nutrition education efforts by other programs, and several other factors. Specific proposals by the presenters included the use of comparative effectiveness studies in numerous sites in four to eight states and the merging of results through appropriate analysis. Following TREND guidelines and writing strategy statements may be helpful in reports provided to funders and in journal papers.

REFERENCES

Abusabha, R., C. Achterberg, J. McKenzie, and D. Torres. 1998. Evaluation of nutrition education in WIC. Evaluation of nutrition education in a supplemental food and nutrition program in New Mexico. *Journal of Family and Consumer Sciences: From Research to Practice* 90(4):98–104.

Anderson, J. V., D. I. Bybee, R. M. Brown, D. F. McLean, E. M. Garcia, M. L. Breer, and B. A. Schillo. 2001. 5 a day fruit and vegetable intervention improves consumption in a low income population. *Journal of the American Dietetic Association* 101(2):195–202.

Bensley, R. J., J. J. Brusk, J. V. Anderson, N. Mercer, J. Rivas, and L. N. Broadbent. 2006. WICHealth.org: Impact of a stages of change-based Internet nutrition education program. *Journal of Nutrition Education & Behavior* 38(4):222–229.

Birmingham, B., J. A. Shultz, and M. Edlefsen. 2004. Evaluation of a five-a-day recipe booklet for enhancing the use of fruits and vegetables in low-income households. *Journal of Community Health* 29(1):45–62.

Block, G., M. Miller, L. Harnack, S. Kayman, S. Mandel, and S. Cristofar. 2000. An interactive CD-ROM for nutrition screening and counseling. *American Journal of Public Health* 90(5):781–785.

Campbell, M. K., E. Carbone, L. Honess-Morreale, J. Heisler-Mackinnon, S. Demissie, and D. Farrell. 2004. Randomized trial of a tailored nutrition education CD-ROM program for women receiving food assistance. *Journal of Nutrition Education & Behavior* 36(2):58–66.

Carroll, J. M., C. Stein, M. Byron, and K. Dutram. 1996. Using interactive multimedia to deliver nutrition education to Maine's WIC clients. *Journal of Nutrition Education* 28(1):19–25.

Cena, E. R., A. B. Joy, K. Heneman, G. Espinosa-Hall, L. Garcia, C. Schneider, P. C. Wooten Swanson, M. Hudes, and S. Zidenberg-Cherr. 2008. Learner-centered nutrition education improves folate intake and food-related behaviors in nonpregnant, low-income women of childbearing age. *Journal of the American Dietetic Association* 108(10):1627–1635.

Chang, M.-W., S. Nitzke, and R. Brown. 2010. Design and outcomes of a mothers in motion behavioral intervention pilot study. *Journal of Nutrition Education & Behavior* 42(3 Suppl.):S11–S21.

Crawford P. B., W. Gosliner, P. Strode, S. E. Samuels, C. Burnett, L. Craypo, and A. K. Yancey. 2004. Walking the talk: Fit WIC wellness programs improve self-efficacy in pediatric obesity prevention counseling. *American Journal of Public Health* 94(9):1480–1485.

Des Jarlais, D. C., C. Lyles, and N. Crepaz. 2004. Improving the reporting quality of nonrandomized evaluations of behavioral and public health intreventions: The TREND statement. *American Journal of Public Health* 94(3):361–366.

Fahrenwald, N. L., J. R. Atwood, S. N. Walker, D. R. Johnson, and K. Berg. 2004. A randomized pilot test of "moms on the move": A physical activity intervention for WIC mothers. *Annals of Behavioral Medicine* 27(2):82–90.

Faith, M. S., R. I. Berkowitz, V. A. Stallings, J. Kerns, M. Storey, and A. J. Stunkard. 2004. Parental feeding attitudes and styles and child body mass index: Prospective analysis of a gene-environment interaction. *Pediatrics* 114(4):e429–436.

Fisher, J. O., and L. L. Birch. 1999. Restricting access to foods and children's eating. *Appetite* 32(3):405–419.

Fisher, J. O., and L. L. Birch. 2002. Eating in the absence of hunger and overweight in girls from 5 to 7 y of age. *American Journal of Clinical Nutrition* 76(1):226–231.

Gerstein, D. E., A. C. Martin, N. Crocker, H. Reed, M. Elfant, and P. Crawford. 2010. Using learner-centered education to improve fruit and vegetable intake in California WIC participants. *Journal of Nutrition Education & Behavior* 42(4):216–224.

Havas, S., K. Treiman, P. Langenberg, M. Ballesteros, J. Anliker, D. Damron, and R. Feldman. 1998. Factors associated with fruit and vegetable consumption among women participating in WIC. *Journal of the American Dietetic Association* 98(10):1141–1148.

Ikeda, J. P., L. Pham, K.-P. Nguyen, and R. A. Mitchell. 2002. Culturally relevant nutrition education improves dietary quality among WIC-eligible Vietnamese immigrants. *Journal of Nutrition Education & Behavior* 34(3):151–158.

Johnson, D. B., D. Birkett, C. Evens, and S. Pickering. 2005. Statewide intervention to reduce television viewing in WIC clients and staff. *American Journal of Health Promotion* 19(6):418–421.

Johnson, D. B., D. Birkett, C. Evens, and S. Pickering. 2006. Promoting family meals in WIC: Lessons learned from a statewide initiative. *Journal of Nutrition Education and Behavior* 38(3):177–182.

Krummel, D., E. Semmens, A. M. MacBride, and B. Fisher. 2010. Lessons learned from the mothers' overweight management study in 4 West Virginia WIC offices. *Journal of Nutrition Education & Behavior* 42(3 Suppl.):S52–S58.

Lee, Y., D. C. Mitchell, H. Smiciklas-Wright, and L. L. Birch. 2001. Diet quality, nutrient intake, weight status, and feeding environments of girls meeting or exceeding recommendations for total dietary fat of the American Academy of Pediatrics. *Pediatrics* 107(6): e95–121.

Michie, S., and C. Abraham. 2004. Interventions to change health behaviours: Evidence-based or evidence-inspired? *Psychology & Health* 19(1):29–49.

Michie, S., C. Abraham, C. Whittington, J. McAteer, and S. Gupta. 2009. Effective techniques in healthy eating and physical activity interventions: A meta-regression. *Health Psychology* 28(6):690–701.

Nestor, B., J. McKenzie, N. Hasan, R. AbuSabha, and C. Achterberg. 2001. Client satisfaction with the nutrition education component of the California WIC program. *Journal of Nutrition Education* 33(2):83–94.

Prochaska, J. O., C. C. DiClemente, and J. C. Norcross. 1992. In search of how people change. Applications to addictive behaviors. *The American Psychologist* 47(9): 1102–1114.

Ritchie, L. D., S. E. Whaley, P. Spector, J. Gomez, and P. B. Crawford. 2010. Favorable impact of nutrition education on California WIC families. *Journal of Nutrition Education and Behavior* 42(3 Suppl.):S2–S10.

Tessaro, I., S. Rye, L. Parker, C. Mangone, and S. McCrone. 2007. Effectiveness of a nutrition intervention with rural low-income women. *American Journal of Health Behavior* 31(1):35–43.

Trepka, M. J., F. L. Newman, F. G. Huffman, and Z. Dixon. 2010. Food safety education using an interactive multimedia kiosk in a WIC setting: Correlates of client satisfaction and practical issues. *Journal of Nutrition Education and Behavior* 42(3):202–207.

USDA/ERS (U.S. Department of Agriculture/Economic Research Service). 2007. *Using Point-of-Purchase Data to Evaluate Local WIC Nutrition Education Interventions: Feasibility Study.* Washington, DC: USDA/ERS. http://hdl.handle.net/10113/32797 (accessed September 16, 2010).

USDA/FNS (U.S. Department of Agriculture/Food and Nutrition Service). 2000. *WIC Nutrition Education Assessment Study Final Report, September 1998.* Alexandria, VA: USDA/FNS.

USDA/FNS. 2001a. *WIC Nutrition Education Demonstration Study: Prenatal Intervention.* Washington, DC: USDA/FNS. http://www.fns.usda.gov/oane/Menu/Published/WIC/FILES/WICNutEdPrenatal.pdf (accessed September 30, 2010).

USDA/FNS. 2001b. *WIC Nutrition Education Demonstration Study: Child Intervention.* Washington, DC: USDA/FNS. http://hdl.handle.net/10113/38348 (accessed September 16, 2010).

USDA/National Agriculture Library. 2006. *WIC Works Resource System: WIC Program Nutrition Education Guidance.* http://www.nal.usda.gov/wicworks/Learning_Center/ntredguidance.pdf (accessed September 24, 2010).

Whaley, S. E., L. D. Ritchie, P. Spector, J. Gomez, and P. B. Crawford. Submitted. Revised WIC food package produces intended behavior change in WIC families. *Journal of Nutrition Education and Behavior*

Whaley, S. E., S. McGregor, L. Jiang, J. Gomez, G. Harrison, and E. Jenks. 2010. A WIC-based intervention to prevent early childhood overweight. *Journal of Nutrition Education and Behavior* 42(3 Suppl.):S47–S51.

Woelfel, M. L., R. AbuSabha, R. Pruzek, H. Stratton, S. G. Chen, and L. S. Edmunds. 2004. Barriers to the use of WIC services. *Journal of the American Dietetic Association* 104(5):736–743.

8

Health Care and Systems Costs, Benefits, and Effectiveness

In opening this session, moderator Barbara Devaney noted that the Special Supplemental Nutrition Program for Women, Infants, and Children (WIC) might affect health care costs in two opposing ways and suggested that the speakers might address these effects. On one hand, WIC may lead to improved dietary and health behaviors that would lead to better health, fewer adverse health outcomes, and reduced health care costs. On the other hand, it is possible that WIC's referrals and improved linkages to the health care system could lead to increased health care utilization and increased health care costs.

During the session, Sally Findley focused on research related to long-term health and system impacts associated with WIC, while Helen Jensen addressed elements of human health risk–benefit assessment and their implications for research.

SUGGESTIONS FOR ASSESSING THE LONG-TERM HEALTH AND SYSTEM IMPACTS ASSOCIATED WITH WIC

Presenter: Sally E. Findley

"Optimistic" Logic Model

Findley presented an "optimistic" logic model for assessing WIC's impact on health care outcomes, an abbreviated version of which is shown in Figure 8-1. On the far right of the figure are the long-term impacts that

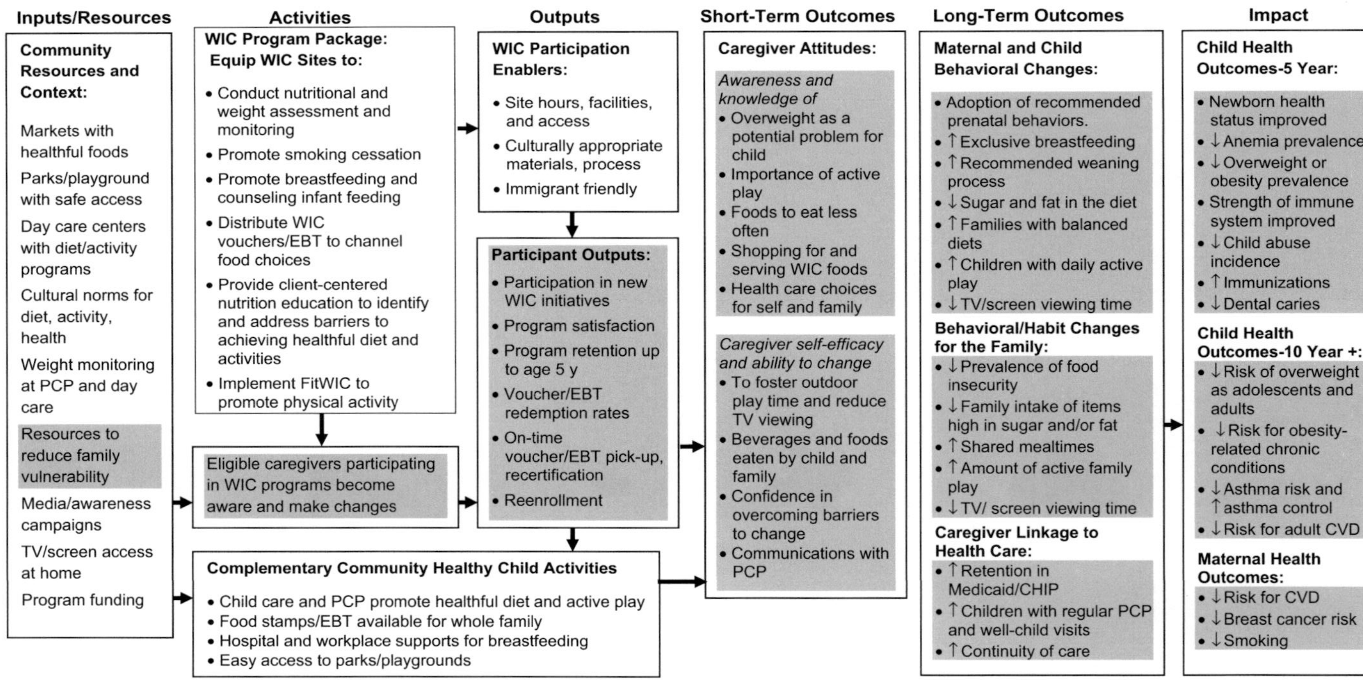

FIGURE 8-1 Abbreviated version of Findley's optimistic logic model for assessing WIC's impact on health care outcomes. Outcomes would be measured to determine the extent to which favorable results have occurred.
NOTE: ↑ = increased; ↓ = decreased; CHIP = Child Health Insurance Program; CVD = cardiovascular disease; EBT = electronic benefit transfer; PCP = primary care provider; TV = television. Fit WIC is a collection of social and environmental strategies to promote healthy weight among children enrolled in WIC.
SOURCE: Findley (2010).

can be anticipated from effective WIC services—in particular, impacts that could affect health care utilization and costs. One purpose of the logic model is to show the causal pathway that links WIC activities (box on left) with these impacts. The intermediary boxes show where changes occur through both short-term changes in caregiver attitudes, such as knowledge about the importance of low fat milk consumption, and increased caregiver self-efficacy. The subsequent long-term outcomes can include maternal and behavioral changes, some of which (e.g., reduced food insecurity) could affect the entire family's health behaviors. The actual child health outcomes appear in the boxes at the far right and are listed as outcomes occurring after 5 years and after 10 or more years.

Considering Impacts Over Time

Rationale

According to Findley, WIC needs studies that document the different time frames over which effects take place. Currently, there are time-sensitive opportunities for 5-year WIC impact assessments that relate to the previous and current WIC food packages, effects of the recession and of changes in insurance coverage pursuant to the Affordable Health Care Act, and linkages with clinical programs seeking to promote patient-centered care. Findley found no studies that have looked at effects of WIC after 5 years. Child health studies, however, show evidence of possible long-term health outcomes of WIC for children, and maternal health studies suggest long-term health benefits for both women and their children (see Box 8-1). Even if the long-term benefits of WIC are fairly small, they could potentially be very large when multiplied over the entire population affected. Evidence of strong long-term consequences could provide additional details needed to extend cost–benefit and cost-effectiveness analyses.

Challenges

Long-term studies pose many challenges, including the tracking of WIC participants over time and difficulties obtaining accurate data on the intensity of and exposure to WIC services for a given mother-child dyad. The optimistic logic model can be used to tease out the possible mechanisms by which the WIC influence might be transmitted over time through sustained behavioral changes.

BOX 8-1
Evidence of Possible Long-Term Health Outcomes of WIC

Children

- Better birth outcomes: reductions in asthma and chronic lung disease (Dietert and Zelikoff, 2008; Fiorino and Brooks, 2009; Oddy et al., 2004)
- Weight gain reductions: reduced chronic disease risk (Franks et al., 2010; Hyppönen et al., 2000; McGillis Bindler, 2007; Van Cleave et al., 2010)
- Maternal smoking cessation: reduced asthma risk (Gold et al.,1999; Morgan, 1998)
- Breastfeeding and nutrition: improved immune system (Chulada et al., 2003; DiGiorgio and Danoff, 2005).
- Breastfeeding and reduced sweet consumption: fewer early childhood dental caries (Lee et al., 2004)
- Improved early childhood health status: better health at later ages (Goran et al., 2003; Lamb et al., 2010; Serdula et al., 1993)

Women

- Dietary changes and weight loss counseling: reduced obesity (Klohe-Lehman et al., 2007; Papas et al., 2009), with potential impact on childhood obesity (Huang et al., 2007)
- Weight gain reductions: reduced gestational and type 2 diabetes risk (Laraia et al., 2010; Nelson et al., 2010)
- Breastfeeding: reduced breast cancer risk (Steube et al., 2009)
- Smoking cessation: reduced lung and heart disease (Roelands et al., 2009)

Potential Research Topics

Child Health

Findley suggested several high-priority research topics concerning the long-term impact of WIC on child health. These include WIC-related exclusive breastfeeding as protection from chronic disorders, the durability of any WIC-related reduction in body mass index through adolescence (e.g., does a decay model describe the findings, or is there evidence of positive synergistic interaction with subsequent interventions?), the effect of WIC participation on health care utilization and costs 5 to 15 years post WIC, and the effect of WIC to age 21 among a cohort followed through the National Children's Study.

Maternal and Family Health

High-priority maternal-health-outcome studies include the effectiveness of WIC interventions during pregnancy to promote lasting behavioral and diet changes among mothers, linkages between changes in the diets of mothers and the diets of their infants and children enrolled in WIC, effects of repeat WIC "doses" of counseling and checks on changes in family diet and activity patterns, changes in health care utilization and costs for WIC mothers (controlling for household economic security and prior chronic conditions), and the effects of co-locating WIC and Healthy Start and Healthy Families programs on maternal health behaviors and outcomes.

Changes in Health Care Utilization

An often overlooked behavioral component of WIC is change in health care utilization. Relatively little attention has been paid to the linkages between WIC and the primary health care system and continuity of care, even though there is much evidence that continuity of care has a positive effect on many preventive behaviors and on chronic disease management (Flores et al., 2005; Groner et al., 2009; Nelson et al., 2005). Kendal and colleagues (2002) have reported increased positive changes in health behavior when WIC is co-located with a managed-care organization.

Research Priorities

First Priority

Findley's number one research priority is a long-term prospective study of WIC versus non-WIC children with a baseline and 5- and 10-year follow-ups, as indicated in Table 8-1.

The child health outcomes would include changes in body mass index, diet and physical activity, television viewing, and health care utilization. The same individuals would be evaluated at each time period. Co-variates to be tracked longitudinally would include the child's family situation, maternal behaviors, participation in Head Start or parenting programs, continuity of care, and neighborhood factors that may contribute to obesity.

The National Children's Study would be the best candidate data set for this research because the study is nationwide; centers will be located

TABLE 8-1 Proposed Design of Prospective Study of WIC Versus Non-WIC Children

	WIC-High Exposure	WIC-Low Exposure	Non-WIC Exposure
Baseline (2010–2011)			
5-Year Follow-Up			
10-Year Follow-Up			

in every state; vanguard sites are already recruiting cohorts; the study will collect extensive details regarding the prenatal situation, the mother's situation, and the child's situation at each point in time; and it will track neighborhood influences for each time period.

Second Priority

Findley's second priority for WIC research is a study to determine the durability of the changes in behavior, food intake, and weight that are achieved among WIC participants with the new WIC package of foods and counseling. Such a study would use upcoming data from the new National Survey of Children's Health (http://www.cdc.gov/nchs/slaits/nsch.htm). It may be possible to include WIC participation variables in the survey instrument, which is still in development. The multi-level and 5-year analysis would include the timing and intensity of WIC participation, qualitative interviews with selected WIC staff and participants, community characteristics, and primary care linkages. A particular focus would be maternal behaviors and maternal and child outcomes.

Third Priority

Findley's third priority addresses the question "How is the WIC message enhanced through coordination with primary care providers?" She described a comparative effectiveness study that would be designed with multiple study arms, one for each type of linkage with a primary health care (PHC) provider: no PHC, PHC for maternal care, PHC for child health care, and joint linkage for maternal and child care. The design could also control for the style of PHC, such as whether the PHC provider offered patient-centered care, shared electronic medical records with WIC, or was co-located with WIC. This study would track WIC retention, behavioral and health outcomes, and health care utilization. Among the methodological concerns are issues relating to the measurement of WIC exposure, the time horizon for impact assessment, the key covariates, and the accurate description of the primary care structure and linkages.

Closing Comments

Findley emphasized that assessing the cost-effectiveness of WIC requires the careful identification of outcomes—both those that are targeted directly and those that may occur over the long term (such as the reduction of obesity, asthma, or diabetes).

PERSPECTIVES ON RISK–BENEFIT ASSESSMENT

Presenter: Helen H. Jensen

In opening her presentation, Jensen pointed out that WIC could be considered a bridge from the food programs to the health system. As shown in Table 8-2, WIC is one of several important food programs of the U.S. Department of Agriculture (USDA). Jensen took the perspective of looking at the risks and benefits relative to programs targeted to mothers, infants, and young children.

Elements of Human Health Risk–Benefit Assessment

The European Food Safety Authority gives the following definition of *benefit*, in the context of a health risk–benefit assessment: "The probability of a positive health effect and/or the probability of a reduction of an adverse health effect in an organism, system, or (sub) population, in reaction to exposure to an agent" (EFSA, 2010, p. 8). This broad definition indicates that WIC research into health benefits should aim to understand the context of the effect, the exposure, the intervention or policy, and the aspect of the program that is having the effect.

The risk–benefit assessment paradigm includes four elements: (1) identification of health effects, both positive and negative; (2) characterization of the health effect (the dose–response assessment; (3) exposure assessment; and (4) benefit characterization. The expected health effects would be examined for the target population. Health effects could be direct or indirect and would include the response to program participation; the response to program parameters, such as benefits and interventions; and the longevity of the response relative to differences in the intensity and duration of exposure and evidence of carryover. Exposure assessment addresses the populations that are reached, the extent of participation of at-risk populations, the duration and intensity of the exposure (e.g., breastfeeding) relative to those populations, and covariates (e.g., labor force participation issues relative to breastfeeding). Careful characterization of benefits is especially important

TABLE 8-2 Budgets for U.S. Department of Agriculture Food Programs, Federal Year 2011

Program	2011 Budget (in millions)
Supplemental Nutrition Assistance Program (SNAP)	$68,207
Child Nutrition Programs	$18,392
Special Supplemental Nutrition Program (WIC)	$7,603

SOURCE: USDA (2010).

for developing a more integrated understanding of relationships among WIC and health outcomes.

Jensen suggested that consideration be given to including three health risks in the WIC research agenda: low birth rate, obesity, and food insecurity. Human health benefits could result from interventions that reduce those adverse effects and enhance positive effects. Cost-effectiveness analysis could investigate the cost-effectiveness of program interventions relative to expenditures across various programs or else provide a comparative assessment of the three kinds of WIC interventions (supplemental food packages, nutrition education, and referrals to health services).

In conducting a comparative risk–benefit assessment, one must identify and consider multiple metrics and recognize that an increase in preventive services may increase health care costs. One also needs to consider the strength of the evidence and uncertainty. Uncertainties increase when examining longer-term associations. Combining risks and benefits in a systematic framework assists in setting priorities. A comparative assessment needs to distinguish substitute activities, complementary activities, and reinforcing activities and determine how best to build on the joint activities in the system.

To improve risk–benefit management decisions, one needs to understand key differences between treatment and prevention activities and determine how best to give value to prevention activities. A question for studies spanning the 1- to 5-year range might be, "What health care costs were saved by early interventions?" Effects need to be considered for individuals and for the household—both in terms of food and in terms of interactions with the health care system.

Implications for Research

In health care, the time horizon requires careful attention, as does the value of longer-term outcomes. The characterization of benefits for various program populations will differ considerably. Cross-program effects (such as concurrent participation in health care, immunizations, and prenatal care) make it especially challenging to distinguish among what is attributable to WIC, associated with WIC, or a product of other health care system interventions.

Jensen called for efforts to establish linkages between WIC interventions and health care utilization and outcomes. In the case of mothers, for example, how do incentives to breastfeed carry over in terms of improvements for the mother and for the household? Common metrics are needed that align with WIC and with related health programs. Finally, she suggested that data are needed on cross-program participation (including the diversity of participants and changing demographics) and the household's exposure to the health care system.

RESPONSE

Discussant: Paul Buescher

In his response, Buescher commented on several issues related to cost studies that were raised during this and other sessions. In particular, he highlighted important types of evaluations, addressed some methodological challenges, and raised some new questions, as summarized below:

- *Evaluations linking administrative data from WIC, Medicaid, and birth certificates* It would be useful to update such evaluations for time periods when the new WIC packages have become available, taking care to improve methods to reduce biases.
- *Linkages between WIC interventions and health care utilization and outcomes* Perhaps many of the positive effects of WIC arise because of WIC's success in helping its participants make use of other appropriate health and social services. Oral health care linkages may be important to address.
- *Long-term impacts of WIC for children, maternal health, and the interaction between WIC and health care* A major challenge here will be accessing and developing appropriate data sources. One advantage of the longitudinal studies suggested earlier by Murphy and Findley would be the possibility of showing that later health care costs decrease substantially, overshadowing initial increases related to higher use of preventive care services.
- *Overcoming potential biases* Huntington and Connell (1994) discuss several flaws in research methods used in studies of cost savings from prenatal care. Buescher said that it is essential to develop methods to address the problem of self-selection bias, for example, because WIC participants may differ from non-participants on unmeasured characteristics.
- *Benefits of WIC for children* More research is needed on this topic, and new data sources are needed to conduct evaluations of this type. Buescher suggested that USDA staff contact the principal investigators of the National Children's Study to ensure that appropriate data are collected to enable research on WIC, including the assessment of the long-term effects of prenatal and child WIC participation.
- *Criteria for judging WIC* Is cost savings an appropriate criterion? WIC participants in North Carolina had higher use of preventive, diagnostic, and curative medical care services, and this was associated with higher costs for Medicaid (Buescher et al., 2003). This may not be a negative outcome, however, if the health care needs of the WIC children on Medicaid were being met better than were those of non-participants.

- *Consideration of income level* Would it be advisable to stratify by income level in new studies of WIC in order to assess differential effects? The positive results of many of the earlier studies were from a time when the income level for Medicaid enrollment was 100 percent of the federal poverty level or less, in contrast to the current level of at least 185 percent of the poverty level.

GROUP DISCUSSION

Moderator: Barbara Devaney

Topics raised during the group discussion included the following:

- One possible prenatal effect of WIC might be a decrease in the percentage of conceptuses lost before about 22 weeks of gestation accompanied by an increase in the number of very-low-birth-weight or preterm infants, for example.
- Consideration of long-term outcomes requires information over a long period of time and is fraught with potential analytic traps. Methods need to be developed to deal with them.
- Oral health care is an example of a primary care linkage with WIC—one that may merit more attention with regard to both maternal and child health.
- A cost–benefit analysis might consider differences in lifetime earnings of WIC recipients; some data sets would allow examination of the issue. Because of the number of variables and the long timeframe, however, it may be more feasible to examine the relationship of WIC participation with early school performance.
- Differences in the diagnosis and treatment of common childhood diseases for WIC and non-WIC children, as were seen in the North Carolina WIC–Medicaid study, could lead to big differences as the children enter school and beyond, and thus may merit study.

SUMMARY OF SUGGESTED RESEARCH TOPICS

The research suggestions made during this session centered on the investigation of long-term impacts of WIC for children, maternal health, and the interaction between WIC and health care. Among the suggested strategies was linking administrative data from WIC, Medicaid, and birth certificates. Methodological issues addressed included the consideration of risks and benefits, potential biases, and clear identification of WIC's role relative to the health outcomes examined.

REFERENCES

Buescher, P. A., S. J. Horton, B. L. Devaney, S. J. Roholt, A. J. Lenihan, J. T. Whitmire, and J. B. Kotch. 2003. Child participation in WIC: Medicaid costs and use of health care services. *American Journal of Public Health* 93(1):145–150.

Chulada, P. C., S. J. Arbes, Jr., D. Dunson, and D. C. Zeldin. 2003. Breast-feeding and the prevalence of asthma and wheeze in children: Analyses from the third National Health and Nutrition Examination Survey, 1988–1994. *Journal of Allergy and Clinical Immunology* 111(2):328–336.

Dietert, R. R., and J. T. Zelikoff. 2008. Early-life environment, developmental immunotoxicology, and the risk of pediatric allergic disease including asthma. *Birth Defects Research. Part B, Developmental and Reproductive Toxicology* 83(6):547–560.

DiGiorgio, L. F., and N. Danoff. 2005. Promoting breastfeeding to mothers in the Special Supplemental Nutrition Program for Women, Infants, and Children. *Journal of the American Dietetic Association* 105(5):716–717.

EFSA (European Food Safety Authority Scientific Committee). 2010. Guidance on human health risk–benefit assessment of food. *European Food Safety Authority Journal* 8(7):1673. http://www.efsa.europa.eu/en/scdocs/doc/1673.pdf (accessed September 9, 2010).

Findley, S. E. 2010. *Suggestions for assessing the long-term health and system impacts associated with the new WIC packages.* Presented at the IOM workshop, Health Impacts: Planning a WIC Research Agenda. Washington, DC: The National Academies Press.

Fiorino, E. K., and L. J. Brooks. 2009. Obesity and respiratory diseases in childhood. *Clinics in Chest Medicine* 30(3):601–608, x.

Flores, G., L. Olson, and S. C. Tomany-Korman. 2005. Racial and ethnic disparities in early childhood health and health care. *Pediatrics* 115(2):e183–e193.

Franks, P. W., R. L. Hanson, W. C. Knowler, M. L. Sievers, P. H. Bennett, and H. C. Looker. 2010. Childhood obesity, other cardiovascular risk factors, and premature death. *New England Journal of Medicine* 362(6):485–493.

Gold, D. R., H. A. Burge, V. Carey, D. K. Milton, T. Platts-Mills, and S. T. Weiss. 1999. Predictors of repeated wheeze in the first year of life: The relative roles of cockroach, birth weight, acute lower respiratory illness, and maternal smoking. *American Journal of Respiratory and Critical Care Medicine* 160(1):227–236.

Goran, M. I., G. D. Ball, and M. L. Cruz. 2003. Obesity and risk of type 2 diabetes and cardiovascular disease in children and adolescents. *Journal of Clinical Endocrinology and Metabolism* 88(4):1417–1427.

Groner, J. A., T. Skybo, L. Murray-Johnson, P. Schwirian, I. Eneli, A. Sternstein, E. Klein, and G. French. 2009. Anticipatory guidance for prevention of childhood obesity: Design of the MOMS project. *Clinical Pediatrics* 48(5):483–492.

Huang, J. S., T. A. Lee, and M. C. Lu. 2007. Prenatal programming of childhood overweight and obesity. *Maternal and Child Health Journal* 11(5):461–473.

Huntington, J., and F. A. Connell. 1994. For every dollar spent—The cost-savings argument for prenatal care. *New England Journal of Medicine* 331(19):1303–1307.

Hyppönen, E., S. M. Virtanen, M. G. Kenward, M. Knip, and H. K. Åkerblom. 2000. Obesity, increased linear growth, and risk of type 1 diabetes in children. *Diabetes Care* 23(12):1755–1760.

Kendal, A. P., A. Peterson, C. Manning, F. Xu, L. J. Neville, and C. Hogue. 2002. Improving the health of infants on Medicaid by collocating special supplemental nutrition clinics with managed care provider sites. *American Journal of Public Health* 92(3): 399–403.

Klohe-Lehman, D. M., J. Freeland-Graves, K. K. Clarke, G. Cai, V. S. Voruganti, T. J. Milani, H. J. Nuss, J. M. Proffitt, and T. M. Bohman. 2007. Low-income, overweight and obese mothers as agents of change to improve food choices, fat habits, and physical activity in their 1-to-3-year-old children. *Journal of the American College of Nutrition* 26(3):196–208.

Lamb, M. M., D. Dabelea, X. Yin, L. G. Ogden, G. J. Klingensmith, M. Rewers, and J. M. Norris. 2010. Early-life predictors of higher body mass index in healthy children. *Annals of Nutrition and Metabolism* 56(1):16–22.

Laraia, B. A., A. M. Siega–Riz, and C. Gundersen. 2010. Household food insecurity is associated with self-reported pregravid weight status, gestational weight gain, and pregnancy complications. *Journal of the American Dietetic Association* 110(5):692–701.

Lee, J. Y., R. G. Rozier, E. C. Norton, J. B. Kotch, and W. F. Vann, Jr. 2004. Effects of WIC participation on children's use of oral health services. *American Journal of Public Health* 94(5):772–777.

McGillis Bindler, R. C. 2007. A cascade of events—Obesity, metabolic syndrome, and type 2 diabetes mellitus in youth. *Nursing Clinics of North America* 42(1):29–42, vi.

Morgan, W. J. 1998. Maternal smoking and infant lung function. Further evidence for an in utero effect. *American Journal of Respiratory and Critical Care Medicine* 158(3): 689–690.

Nelson, C. S., S. M. Higman, C. Sia, E. McFarlane, L. Fuddy, and A. K. Duggan. 2005. Medical homes for at-risk children: Parental reports of clinician–parent relationships, anticipatory guidance, and behavior changes. *Pediatrics* 115(1):48–56.

Nelson, S. M., P. Matthews, and L. Poston. 2010. Maternal metabolism and obesity: Modifiable determinants of pregnancy outcome. *Human Reproduction Update* 16(3):255–275.

Oddy, W. H., J. L. Sherriff, N. H. de Klerk, G. E. Kendall, P. D. Sly, L. J. Beilin, K. B. Blake, L. I. Landau, and F. J. Stanley. 2004. The relation of breastfeeding and body mass index to asthma and atopy in children: A prospective cohort study to age 6 years. *American Journal of Public Health* 94(9):1531–1537.

Papas, M. A., K. M. Hurley, A. M. Quigg, S. E. Oberlander, and M. M. Black. 2009. Low-income, African American adolescent mothers and their toddlers exhibit similar dietary variety patterns. *Journal of Nutrition Education and Behavior* 41(2):87–94.

Roelands, J., M. G. Jamison, A. D. Lyerly, and A. H. James. 2009. Consequences of smoking during pregnancy on maternal health. *Journal of Women's Health* 18(6):867–872.

Serdula, M. K., D. Ivery, R. J. Coates, D. S. Freedman, D. F. Williamson, and T. Byers. 1993. Do obese children become obese adults? A review of the literature. *Preventive Medicine* 22(2):167–177.

Stuebe, A. M., W. C. Willett, F. Xue, and K. B. Michels. 2009. Lactation and incidence of premenopausal breast cancer: A longitudinal study. *Archives of Internal Medicine* 169(15):1364–1371.

USDA (U.S. Department of Agriculture). 2010. *FY 2011 Budget Summary and Annual Performance Plan*. Washington, DC: USDA. http://www.obpa.usda.gov/budsum/FY11budsum.pdf (accessed September 10, 2010).

Van Cleave, J., S. L. Gortmaker, and J. M. Perrin. 2010. Dynamics of obesity and chronic health conditions among children and youth. *Journal of the American Medical Association* 303(7):623–630.

9

The Reach of WIC

At the outset of this session, the workshop moderator, Gail Harrison, mentioned that the planning committee struggled with a title for the session. Its intent was to look at the overall influence of the Special Supplemental Nutrition Program for Women, Infants, and Children (WIC) on families and on society more broadly. Then session moderator Jackson Sekhobo offered brief remarks about why research on the reach of WIC is especially important at the local and state levels. Data are used by states for funding decisions, for which the key questions may be whether a program is effective and whether it contributes to the core mission of the agency. He emphasized the following four points:

1. From a state perspective, the most widely used indicators for WIC are participation rates among eligible persons and redemption rates among participants. Participation rates are useful for various stakeholders, including advocates and legislators.
2. Because states are expected to engage in program outreach and marketing, they must demonstrate success in penetrating hard-to-reach WIC-eligible populations.
3. Participation rates, redemption rates, and administrative expenses are all used in the federal funding formula for the allocation of funds to states, with more dollars directed to states with higher participation rates.
4. In terms of the Office of Management and Budget's definition of an effective federally funded program, WIC can be considered effective because it reaches large numbers of eligible low-income

persons, it has been associated with improved health outcomes, and the increase in the cost of the food package over time has been less than the rate of inflation.

The challenge given to the presenters, Susan Bartlett and Loren Bell, and the discussant, Zoë Neuberger, was to address new ways of documenting the reach of WIC given various changes that have occurred within WIC, the impending health care reform, and the changing demographics of the WIC-eligible population.

PERSPECTIVES

Presenter: Susan Bartlett[1]

Useful Information for Policymakers

A group at Abt Associates used a series of questions to develop recommendations for a WIC research agenda. Starting with the question "What information would be most useful to policymakers?" the group laid out two broad topics for discussion: (1) "How well is WIC working now?" and (2) "How could WIC work better?" Under the first topic, the questions were centered on whether WIC is necessary, sufficient, benign, and cost-effective. The second topic focused on ways to increase WIC's effectiveness in achieving objectives and ways to remove or reduce unintended adverse consequences.

Concerning the issue of whether to try to measure the overall impact of WIC, the group identified various reasons not to try, including the difficulty—perhaps impossibility—of measuring the impact accurately and the high level of support for WIC. However, it also identified a number of reasons to try to make such measurements, such as determining whether there are deleterious effects, identifying variations among subgroups that could lead to program improvements, and providing evidence to support increased program funding.

Potential Research Topics

The group's discussions led to the identification of four research domains: (1) WIC participation, (2) a logic model for effects, (3) potential improvements to the program, and (4) experimental studies to investigate impacts. Each of these is discussed briefly below.

[1]Bartlett credited the contributions of many of her colleagues at Abt Associates.

WIC Participation

A series of focus groups could help provide a better understanding of the characteristics of WIC participants and eligible non-participants. For example, compared with non-participants, are WIC participants more or less needy, motivated, or faced with problems related to time management or substance abuse? Three sets of focus groups were suggested, which would consist of (1) eligible non-participants, (2) late enrollees (pregnant women in their third trimester, postpartum women, and mothers of older infants and children), and (3) women who have left WIC. Such focus groups could offer insights on such topics as women's reasons for not participating, their understandings of nutrition, the difficulties they encountered while on WIC, and their view of the foods provided. This information, in turn, could be used to generate hypotheses for further study.

Another approach to understanding participation would be to compare either the dietary intake of those who leave the program with that of those who stay or else the dietary intake of early entrants versus late entrants. This type of study would require prospective data on diet, some of which might be collected as part of the initial certification interview.

Logic Model

The concept of a logic model had been presented earlier in the workshop by Findley (see Chapter 8). A logic model for WIC would map out the pathways linking interventions with specific outcomes. Studies would be designed to test specific linkages in the model. Among the linkages that would be useful to investigate are interventions associated with the length of gestation; voucher redemptions; the consumption of WIC foods by participants and other household members; and changes that occur between the times of certification and recertification in such measures as weight status, iron status, and dietary patterns. The results would provide suggestive rather than definitive evidence about effects.

Potential Program Improvements

This research domain would address potential changes to WIC that could improve participants' behaviors in the areas of diet, breastfeeding, smoking cessation, and various aspects of preventive care. One suggestion was to consider interventions that have been effective in these domains outside of WIC, such as home visits.

Bartlett identified several approaches for addressing possible ways to improve participants' behaviors. Focus groups involving WIC participants could identify what it might take for them to change, and focus groups with local WIC staff could identify the barriers to change that the staff have observed when working with participants. Bartlett suggested a number of "outside-the box" possibilities. These ideas included providing large (e.g., $100) vouchers for fruits and vegetables, offering new mothers a choice between formula and diapers, charging a co-payment for formula, providing vouchers to be used in fast-food restaurants for WIC-approved foods, and obtaining celebrity endorsements.

Experimental Studies

Abt Associates is conducting a randomized controlled trial that is examining the effects of enhanced breastfeeding support, especially more intensive contacts soon after birth. Pilot studies could be conducted to test some of the "outside the box" ideas mentioned above. To test the importance of the WIC food packages, for example, pilot studies could compare the results of providing WIC vouchers (or WIC electronic benefit transfer [EBT] cards), cash, and Supplemental Nutrition Assistance Program (SNAP) benefits.

THE NEW FOOD PACKAGE

Presenter: Loren Bell

In his presentation, Bell briefly described research being conducted by the Altarum Institute, focusing on two studies designed to examine the effects of the new food package on food purchasing behavior and on small stores. He then identified future research needs related to those topics and to broader issues.

Overview of Current Research

The new WIC food package will be a major focus of the Altarum Institute's food assistance and nutrition activities over the next several years. It is viewed as the most dramatic change to WIC since WIC's inception. The new package aligns nutrition messages with opportunities to purchase healthful foods, it provides opportunities for participants to change their behaviors, and it offers retail food stores the opportunity to make changes that could affect the communities' access to more healthful foods. Box 9-1 highlights some of the topics and questions that are being addressed by Altarum Institute programs. Brief descriptions of two of those programs, the food purchasing pattern study and the small store participation study, follow.

BOX 9-1
Current Focus of Altarum Institute's WIC Food Package Studies

- *Client choices and behaviors*: What foods are clients selecting?
- *Redemption patterns*: Are clients purchasing all the new foods?
- *Retail compliance*: Have stores adjusted inventory?
- *Food quality*: Are the products being offered desirable to clients?
- *Built environment*[a]: Does the new food package make healthful foods available to all?

[a]In this case, the built environment refers to physical aspects of the neighborhood such as grocery stores, sidewalks, and public transportation.

Food Purchasing Pattern Study

The analysis of the food purchasing patterns of WIC clients uses point-of-sale purchasing data matched with WIC demographic data. The study is being conducted in a single state (Wisconsin) and includes mostly chain or major independent stores. Universal Product Code (UPC) data are being linked with WIC issuance records in order to obtain demographic profiles of the purchasing patterns. The patterns are being analyzed at four points in time—prior to implementation and at 6, 12, and 18 months after implementation—and focus groups are being used to examine behaviors.

Small Store Study

The second study is assessing the effect of the new WIC food package on small store participation in WIC. It is examining many factors, including the pre- and post-implementation participation of small rural and urban stores in four states (Pennsylvania, New Hampshire, Wisconsin, and Colorado); the factors contributing to ongoing participation or dropping out; policy decisions, implementation strategies, and wholesale networks; and the availability of new foods. Investigators are making inventories of food availability and freshness, and they are conducting interviews with store owners or managers and with state staff.

Future Research Needs

Based in part on preliminary findings from the two categories of ongoing studies described above, Bell identified the following research needs.

Client Purchasing and Behaviors

- Changes in redemption patterns over the next 2 years;
- Differences in redemption patterns between clients who have been on WIC before and clients new to WIC;
- Seasonal variances in the purchase of fruits and vegetables;
- The effect of store inventory on redemption patterns;
- Factors related to food availability for minority populations;
- Family influences and other factors that affect clients' food purchase decisions;
- Relationships of the WIC food package with grocer compliance, overcharges, and substitutions;
- The economic effect of new WIC sales on the built environment; and
- The effect of the volume of sales on the built environment.

Small Stores

- Effects of the new WIC food package on the availability of healthful foods for inner city and rural families not on WIC;
- Extent to which retail stores will value WIC and continue program participation;
- Types of small stores that are successful in maintaining or growing WIC business; and
- Long-term effects of the new WIC food package on store inventory decisions.

Closing Remarks

In closing, Bell offered several thoughts on WIC's reach. WIC has the potential to have a significant economic and social impact on public health efforts to fight childhood obesity. Ongoing studies are needed to measure influencing factors and changes. EBT will provide significant opportunities for studies and the collection of new food purchasing data. Finally, WIC must be careful to examine the effect of changes, such as the new food package, on minority populations that are dependent on small stores, particularly with respect to access to healthful foods.

RESPONSE

Discussant: Zoë Neuberger

To set the stage for her remarks, Neuberger explained that the Center on Budget and Policy Priorities is a nonprofit public policy institute that examines various policies with a particular focus on how they may affect low- and moderate-income households. She then spoke about funding for WIC, foods with extra ingredients, the responsiveness of WIC to the economic situation, and a planning process to synthesize and disseminate findings from WIC research.

Funding for WIC

WIC is a discretionary program, not an entitlement program. This means that people eligible for benefits will receive them only if sufficient funds are available. Since 1997, there has been a commitment to provide enough federal funds for WIC so that all eligible applicants can be served. A key reason for conducting research related to WIC is to assess WIC's effectiveness, because evidence of its effectiveness could help maintain this commitment. The likely future budget environment makes a strong research base especially important.

Neuberger emphasized that budget projections for the U.S. national debt under current policies indicate clearly that the nation is on an unsustainable path (see Figure 9-1) and that changes must be made to address the debt. Likely changes include decreases in overall federal spending, especially in discretionary spending.

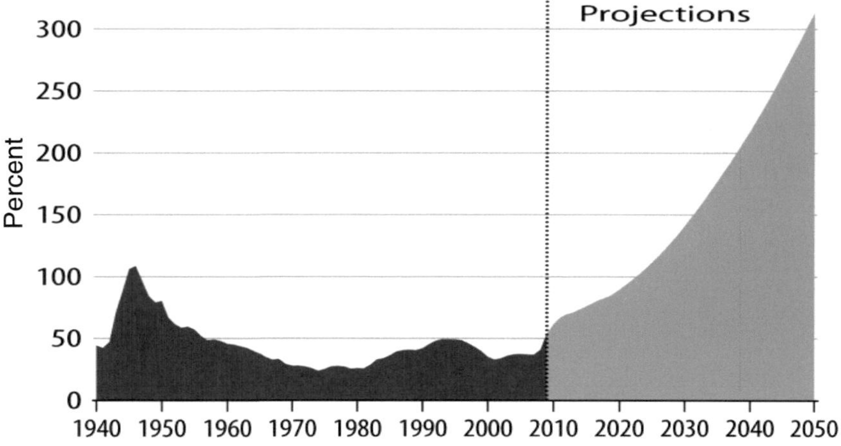

FIGURE 9-1 U.S. national debt as a share of the gross domestic product, 1940–2050.
NOTE: CBPP = Center on Budget and Policy Priorities.
SOURCE: CBPP (2010).

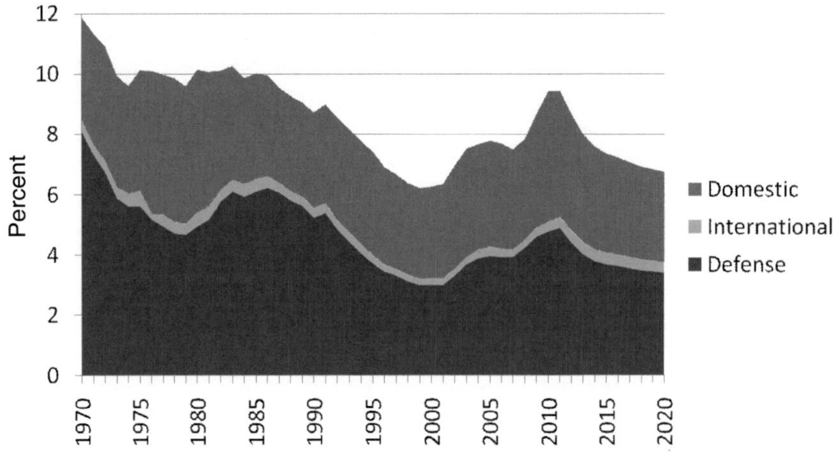

FIGURE 9-2 U.S. discretionary spending as a percentage of the gross domestic product, 1970–2020.
SOURCE: Center on Budget and Policy Priorities (CBPP), based on the Congressional Budget Office's re-estimate of the President's 2011 budget. CBPP adjusted domestic discretionary spending to include Pell grants, which the President proposed to reclassify as mandatory spending

WIC is part of the discretionary spending portion of the budget. In Figure 9-2, WIC is included in the medium-gray section at the top, which represents the domestic discretionary spending portion of the budget. It is worth noting that, based on the administration's budget and forecasts, very substantial decreases in domestic discretionary spending have been projected (a 14 percent decrease between 2005 and 2020). It is anticipated that this will result in increased scrutiny on how WIC spends its funds and an increased need to demonstrate that WIC funds are spent effectively and lead to clearly defined benefits.

Functional Ingredients

Increasingly in the food marketplace, food producers add "functional ingredients"[2] to their foods, and the producers generally charge higher prices for foods with these added ingredients. This practice poses a dilemma for WIC, which needs to decide whether to provide such foods. Currently, the Food and Drug Administration looks at the safety of the added ingredients but does not assess their benefits.

[2]The term *functional ingredients* is used for ingredients that are *claimed* to have health and nutritional benefits.

The Center on Budget and Policy Priorities favors the establishment of a process for assessing such added ingredients. Bills pending in Congress would do this using a two-step process: First, a methodology and framework for assessing the ingredients would be developed, and then the methodology would be applied to assess ingredients that USDA determines warrant review. Neuberger stated that this work should be done with dedicated funding rather than using the funds already allocated for WIC research.

Program Responsiveness to the Economic Situation

WIC participation has been growing about twice as fast as usual during this economic downturn. Based on unemployment rates and increases in poverty and food insecurity, however, the Center on Budget and Policy Priorities had actually expected WIC participation to increase at a much faster rate. Furthermore, the 9 percent growth in WIC participation since the start of the recession is far less than the 47 percent growth in participation that SNAP has experienced over the same period. Neuberger acknowledged that many components affect these numbers; but she said that the magnitude of the disparity in the growth of participation in WIC and SNAP calls for study of the reasons for the difference.

Synthesis and Dissemination of Research Findings

Neuberger's top research priority would be to build mechanisms into the planning process for synthesizing and disseminating WIC research findings. She considers such an effort to be essential to making the results of the research useful to others. In developing the approach, careful attention needs to be given to the many different WIC stakeholders and to how the findings can be presented in forms that will be useful to them.

GROUP DISCUSSION

Moderator: Jackson P. Sekhobo

Many attendees participated in a wide-ranging discussion. Points raised about the research agenda are summarized below.

- *Factors to consider* When conducting studies, it would be useful to consider the following, whenever applicable:
  - o Regional and cultural differences.
  - o Choices that states have made regarding allowed foods, split

tender for fruits and vegetables (i.e., with a split tender, WIC participants may combine cash or other legal tender with their fruit and vegetable vouchers when purchasing allowed fruits and vegetables). The U.S. Department of Agriculture (USDA) is making a database available regarding state policies before and after the change in the food package.
  - The degree to which stores adhere to rules.
  - The interface of WIC with other programs.
  - The various factors, including the value of individual food packages, that affect eligible women's decision about whether or not to participate in WIC.

- *WIC participation* In investigations of WIC participation, it would be useful to have information about the structure of WIC and WIC's degree of dependency on and access to in-kind contributions (e.g., facilities and services provided by health departments). It is worth noting that WIC coverage rates[3] for children have not increased even though the total number of children served by WIC has increased.
- *Redemption data* Because difficulties arise when researchers attempt to obtain access to detailed WIC redemption data, strategies are needed to overcome concerns about confidentiality. One approach may be the application of algorithms that hide identifying personal data when obtaining data on WIC food purchases.
- *Realistic expectations* In view of the relatively small amount of nutrition education and food that participants receive, researchers need to be cautious regarding setting expectations that are too high. A sizable amount of participants' food may actually come from the private food assistance system (e.g., food pantries).
- *Partnerships* Research on how to effectively broaden partnerships would be useful. Beneficial partnerships could include various organizations and stakeholders in the community. Among those mentioned were school nutrition directors, vendors, and those involved with specialty crops.
- *Audiences* People and groups who could benefit from receiving information about WIC research findings include researchers, program administrators, congressional offices, and the media. The key to disseminating the research is to plan ahead for clear communications that use different types of synthesis and dissemination in order to meet the widely differing needs of these audiences. Atten-

[3]The term *WIC coverage rates* refers to the percentage of eligible persons who participate in WIC.

tion should be paid to the dissemination of findings *within* WIC as well as to the audiences mentioned by Neuberger. Receiving such information could affect the attitudes of vendors toward being WIC partners, for example.

SUMMARY OF SUGGESTED RESEARCH TOPICS

Among the many research topics suggested during this session were WIC participation and responsiveness to the nation's financial situation, various applications of the logic model to link interventions with outcomes, ways to have a positive effect on behaviors, the value of the WIC food packages, redemption patterns, the use of the EBT system in tracking food purchases, factors affecting food availability in different settings and for different racial and ethnic groups, and strengthening partnerships. There was a call to develop a plan, at the onset of the research agenda, for the synthesis and dissemination of research findings.

REFERENCE

CBPP (Center on Budget and Policy Priorities). 2010. *The Right Target: Stabilize the Federal Debt*. Washington, DC: CBPP. http://www.cbpp.org/cms/index.cfm?fa=view&id=3049 (accessed September 21, 2010).

10

Closing Session: Wrap-Up and Methodological Issues and Data Considerations

The final session of the workshop included summaries of key points made during the eight sessions, two presentations related to methodological issues and data considerations, an open discussion, and a closing statement from the chair.

HIGHLIGHTS OF PREVIOUS SESSIONS

Presenters: Workshop Moderators

Each moderator presented a brief summary that focused on the research priorities identified in his or her session. Unless indicated otherwise, the research topics are not listed by order of priority in the session summaries. In no instance do they represent group consensus.

Birth Outcomes

Gail G. Harrison

A key message, said Harrison, was to "put the 'W' back in WIC"—that is, focus research on the preconceptional and interconceptional periods. She mentioned biases that are linked with studies of the effects of the Special Supplemental Nutrition Program for Women, Infants, and Children (WIC) on low birth weight and prematurity and the probability that WIC would have a small impact on those outcomes. Maternal health may be viewed as a pathway to improved outcomes for the baby, such as size at birth that is appropriate for gestational age, and the mother. Thought needs to be given to methods for studying how WIC interventions can affect the woman's risk of such outcomes as gestational diabetes and obesity, and especially how WIC could help reduce risks during the first pregnancy. Currently, the interconceptional period provides an opportunity to conduct research on how WIC can influence maternal health and behaviors. Another key message was that researchers should study long-term health outcomes.

Suggested methods for studying birth outcomes included collaboration with the National Children's Study and setting priorities with the goal of gaining the greatest benefit from the research. One way to gain benefit would be to focus on women with prior adverse outcomes or on communities with marked disparities. In a study of relationships of pregnancy outcomes with vitamin D intakes, for example, one could select, as subjects, women at risk for vitamin D deficiency because of dark skin color or lack of exposure to sunlight. Harrison closed her summary by showing selected slides used by the presenters (also see Chapter 2) and reemphasizing the following types of studies:

1. Observational studies on the effect of interconceptional nutrition on birth and long-term child health outcomes.
2. Nutritional intervention studies that begin at interconception.
3. Nutritional research that focuses on women's health before, between, and beyond pregnancy.
4. Studies designed to examine the effects of interventions to reduce preconceptional smoking and obesity, to achieve prenatal weight gain that falls within Institute of Medicine recommendations, and to support breastfeeding.

Overweight and Obesity

Patricia B. Crawford

Obesity has become the foremost health problem of children, said Crawford, and WIC is well positioned to address the problem. A number of risk factors for obesity have been identified, and they are applicable to the diverse population served by WIC. The speakers agreed that studies should focus on messages aimed at reducing those risk factors, and they agreed on study design. In particular, the speakers proposed a multi-stage approach that would involve many community partners as messengers. The first step would be to conduct formative research to develop the preventive messages and to consider the context in which they will be received. The process would include selecting the message that has the most promise for reducing the risk of obesity and also the least potential for harm. Other steps include determining the target behaviors and other positive effects they might have, carrying out the intervention, and examining the fidelity of the intervention. For the types of studies discussed, outcome measures would be behavior changes, not changes in body mass index. Crawford gave the example of developing and testing messages to reduce the excessive consumption of sugar-sweetened beverages.

With respect to Whitaker's mention of the value of working with the messenger as well as addressing the message, Crawford said that her studies indicate that working with the messenger can change the way he or she imparts the message and how the message is received. Adding to the speakers' emphasis on the use of a coordinated community approach and on expanding communication with such other partners as Head Start and pediatricians, Crawford said that it would be very appropriate to include other partners as well.

Breastfeeding

Miriam Labbok

After briefly discussing what is already known about breastfeeding and should therefore be excluded from research priorities (breastfeeding benefits, adverse effects of formula distribution, the importance of no formula during the first month after delivery, a continuum of sensitive individualized breastfeeding care), Labbok first focused on the research topic emphasized during the session on breastfeeding, that is, staffing issues related to peer counselors (their training, competencies, and roles) and lactation consultants and their effects on breastfeeding outcomes. The research would benefit from a phased approach with concurrent elements and program monitoring. Ecological and qualitative studies should be included to identify the issues that need to be studied quantitatively and to gain a better understanding of what had been learned. Perhaps the central piece of research would be group randomized controlled trials that address the peer counseling questions.

Labbok also mentioned three breastfeeding-related research topics that emerged strongly during discussion periods: (1) methods to achieve continuity of care and linkages to the health-care system; (2) perceptions and use of the new WIC food packages and key data needed to examine this issue; and (3) measures to address the inverted economic pressures that the provision of formula causes, perhaps starting with the testing of generic labeling of WIC-provided formula. She encouraged the U.S. Department of Agriculture to consider them for the WIC research agenda as well.

Food Insecurity and Hunger

Maureen Black

Black began her summary by reminding the audience that there are more poor households now than when WIC started and by restating Weill's question, "Is WIC a public health program or an anti-hunger program or an anti-poverty program?" After emphasizing the national importance of reducing food insecurity, its serious consequences for the population served by WIC, and WIC's key role in reducing disparities early in life, Black spoke about the importance of considering the multiple pathways that connect food insecurity with children's well-being. Promising research topics raised during the food insecurity session include the following:

1. Does WIC reduce the likelihood of food insecurity?
2. What effect does WIC have on families that are food insecure?
3. Does WIC affect the stress associated with food insecurity?
4. Does WIC reduce the effects of food insecurity on outcomes?

In examining associations among food insecurity, access to WIC, and WIC's effects on children, it may be useful to consider Frongillo's stress elimination model, compensation model, and buffering model.

Black ended by reiterating Neuberger's concern about how the growing national deficit may lead to efforts to reduce funding for WIC, which could have serious consequences for the nation's children.

Dietary Intake and Nutritional Status

Barbara Devaney

According to Devaney, the basic general question from the session was, "Does WIC participation lead to better diets for women, infants and children?" Specific research priorities proposed during the session included the following:

1. The effect of the new food package on breastfeeding and the timing of complementary feeding.
2. Comparative studies of the consumption of foods provided in the WIC food packages among different groups and under different conditions: specifically, by WIC participants and non-participants at the present time, and by WIC participants prior to and following implementation of the new WIC food packages. Data from the National Health and Nutrition Examination surveys could be used

for these purposes and also to compare nutrient intakes pre- and post-implementation.

Useful data collection and evaluation efforts were identified:

1. Expansion of the types of WIC administrative data to be used for evaluation purposes to include voucher redemption data and certification/recertification data;
2. The use of the administrative data for longitudinal analyses as well as for cross-sectional analyses; and
3. A periodic national survey of WIC participants (and perhaps of non-participants), which, if it had been initiated earlier, would have provided data to answer many of the research questions raised during this workshop.

Nutrition Education

Shannon E. Whaley

Whaley began by saying that a considerable amount is known about nutrition education in WIC and that evidence shows that nutrition education can lead to behavior change. She then said, however, that new data collection strategies are needed to study the effects of the nutrition education that WIC provides. One useful approach would be more consistent reporting of evaluations using non-randomized designs to allow datasets from small studies to be merged.

Using information from the nutrition education session, Whaley proposed a three-step nutrition education research agenda:

1. Conduct qualitative or survey work on how nutrition education is being delivered by WIC across the nation.
2. Determine the outcome measures of highest interest and greatest relevance. What is it that participants want to learn? For example, would obesity prevention messages be of highest priority, and would the messages be meaningful to WIC mothers post partum?
3. Study the comparative effectiveness of various approaches, including, for example, a group approach, a one-on-one approach, an online approach, and a social networking approach. Participants should be assigned to a strategy, probably through the random assignment of WIC sites. The research plan would include delivering the education using the specified approaches, measuring the outcomes, and replicating the studies at different sites.

In addition, Whaley suggested carrying out studies to determine which nutrition education strategies will be most effective for participants who must change the way they shop for WIC foods because of the transition from vouchers to the electronic benefits transfer system.

Health Care and Systems Costs, Benefits, and Effectiveness

Barbara Devaney

Devaney suggested that the logic model presented by Findley (see Chapter 8) was very comprehensive and could provide a useful approach for examining the various research priorities suggested in *all* the workshop's sessions. In conducting health risk–benefit assessment, Jensen had emphasized that careful attention should be given to identifying and characterizing health effects, to assessing dose–response relationships, and characterizing benefits. Devaney said that the key message was to carefully determine which health outcomes should be investigated.

After considering the presentations by Findley and Jensen and the response by Beuscher, Devaney identified the following research priorities related to health care and systems costs, benefits, and effectiveness:

- Analyses of WIC's long-term (5-year and 10-year) effects on such aspects of children's health as relationships among breastfeeding, body mass index, health care utilization, and cost, perhaps using data from the National Survey of Children's Health;
- Analyses concerning maternal health, such as relationships among dietary changes, weight loss counseling, and obesity and between gestational weight gain and the risk of type 2 diabetes; and
- Updating of some of the early WIC evaluations using more types of administrative data and improved statistical methods.

The Reach of WIC

Jackson P. Sekhobo

Sekhobo emphasized that research on the reach of WIC should collect information related to how well WIC is meeting its mission of providing supplemental foods, nutrition education, and referrals to its clients—that is, to pregnant women, breastfeeding and non-breastfeeding postpartum women, and to infants and children up to the age of 5 years. In order to claim that WIC is having beneficial effects on health, it is essential to document that WIC is reaching people, especially through nutrition education. Documenting the reach of WIC might make it possible to determine the proportion of the population-based health improvements that can be attributed to WIC for WIC-eligible populations.

Two overarching research questions were highlighted by Bartlett: (1) How well is WIC working? and (2) How can WIC work better? To address these broad issues, a number of specific research topics were suggested during the session, including analyses of WIC participation, potential improvements to the program, evaluation of the new food package, determination of the benefits and drawbacks of expensive ingredients added to infant formulas, and evaluation of the impact of other public assistance programs (such as the Supplemental Nutrition Assistance Program (SNAP) on participation in WIC. Useful methods that were identified include the REAIM (Reach, Efficacy, Adoption, Implementation, and Maintenance) model for evaluation research and the application of the logic model for effects. Research on the effects of the new food package on redemption would benefit from the use of a pending database that lists state policies before and after the introduction of the new food packages.

METHODOLOGICAL ISSUES AND DATA CONSIDERATIONS

Dietary and Nutrition-Related Issues

Presenter/Discussant: Philip Gleason

Two major challenges in studying the dietary and nutrition-related impacts of WIC are (1) determining how best to measure key outcomes (dietary intake, food insecurity/hunger, biomarkers of nutritional status, and anthropometric outcomes such as body mass index and obesity) and (2) developing a study design that can account for participants' selection into WIC.

Measurement

Measurement issues include identifying the best method to use, deciding on the timing of the reference period, and determining the amount of time required for WIC services to influence outcomes. The measurement of dietary intake typically depends upon 24-hour recalls, which are reports of intake over one particular day rather than a subject's usual intake and which may be subject to misreporting. Using methods developed at Iowa State University and the National Cancer Institute, usual nutrient intake can be estimated for groups if at least two 24-hour recalls are available for a subsample of the population. Estimating the usual food intake is more challenging and may require at least 2 days of recalls for the entire sample. Regression analyses can be used to estimate the effect of WIC on mean usual intake, but they cannot be used to estimate WIC's impact on measures of the distribution of usual intake (such as the proportion of participants with inadequate intake of a particular nutrient).

Timing may be especially important in evaluating such outcomes as the change in iron status (which requires sufficient information about WIC participation over time) and food insecurity (for which the reference period is 12 months).

Study Design

When selecting among feasible design options, researchers should be careful to take both selection bias and representativeness into account. The options that compare WIC participants with some set of non-participants include random assignment and four non-experimental designs: (1) regression discontinuity, (2) comparison group, (3) instrumental variables, and (4) fixed effects.

Random assignment It is likely that random-assignment studies of WIC will only be possible on a small scale. Possible studies include the different approaches to nutrition education mentioned earlier, isolated situations of oversubscription, and the testing of aspects of WIC policy.

Regression discontinuity Regression discontinuity compares people who are just below the income eligibility threshold with those who are just above it. This design requires using the measure of income that is used by the program rather than survey data. Although it provides an unbiased estimate of the impact of WIC, it is not necessarily applicable to the WIC participants with the most need.

Comparison group The comparison-group design usually compares WIC participants with income-eligible non-participants. This design can be applied to groups of the neediest WIC participants, but it has a major drawback in that it is impossible to know if the analysis has accounted for all the non-observable differences between the two groups.

Instrumental variable The instrumental-variables approach uses comparison groups whose participation decision was based on a factor that is strongly correlated with WIC participation but cannot be directly related to the outcome, such as distance of residence from the WIC clinic. Although the method is a sound one, it often has low external validity; and researchers attempting to use instrumental variables to estimate the impact of WIC have generally concluded that they were unable to identify an instrument that works well.

Fixed effects The fixed-effects approach uses variation in WIC participation across time or across siblings within a family, or both, to estimate impacts. Among its disadvantages are a lack of control for unobserved factors that change over time and a lack of sufficiently detailed longitudinal data about participation over time and outcomes.

Conclusions

Selection bias is a particular problem for WIC research. Because the most rigorous designs are likely to have limited external validity, Gleason recommended that the research agenda rely on multiple methods. Timing issues are especially important to consider in studying WIC, in large part because participants' status changes frequently, some outcomes may require that interventions occur over an extended period, and some long-term outcomes are of interest. Large-scale longitudinal data on both WIC participants and non-participants would be especially helpful.

Perinatal Issues

Presenter/Discussant: Theodore Joyce

This presentation by Joyce included a critique of recent studies with large sample sizes that used administrative data, and it provided examples of the four non-experimental study designs described by Gleason (see the preceding section). In his critiques, Joyce emphasized four points:

1. WIC research requires observational studies.
2. Large studies are not necessarily better than smaller ones.
3. The magnitude of the effect must be both plausible and clinically meaningful.
4. Sound research requires appropriate outcomes with confirmatory evidence of causal pathways.

Comparison Group Studies

A large study conducted in Washington state (El-Bastawissi et al., 2007) reported that the rate of preterm births among WIC mothers was 2.7 percentage points lower than the rate among non-WIC mothers, but there was no difference in the rate of low birth weights among full-term babies. Furthermore, the investigators reported that WIC was protective for those who enrolled late in pregnancy (which Joyce pointed out is a measure of inadequate prenatal care). Joyce considered the difference to be implausible and suggestive of gestational age bias (see Chapter 2).

A large study conducted in Florida (Gueorguieva et al., 2009) used redeemed food vouchers to measure the intensity of WIC participation. The researchers found that a 10 percent increase in participation intensity was accompanied by a modest 2.5 percent decrease in small-for-gestational-age births. The matching algorithm was sophisticated, and Joyce considered the outcome to be appropriate and the findings plausible.

Instrumental Variables

Joyce provided the following hypothetical example to illustrate the use of an instrumental variable to simulate a randomized experiment:

> In state X, prenatal WIC funds were depleted several months before the end of the fiscal year. Thus, the eligible pregnant women who conceived near the end of fiscal year would be unable to enroll early. Assuming that the month of depletion is known, this change in funding would provide a natural experiment that would allow investigators to compare outcomes of pregnant women before and after the cutoff of funds.

Using the instrumental variables approach, Figlio et al. (2009) compared rates of low birth weight among women who were marginally income eligible before federal income reporting requirements were made stricter with women who were marginally income eligible after the change. These investigators reported what Joyce considered to be an implausibly large decrease—13 percentage points—in low birth weight among the mothers who met the threshold compared with those who were above it.

Fixed Effects

Joyce offered two examples of the application of fixed effects that used discordant pairs of infants, one of whom was born while the mother was on WIC and the other born when the mother was not. Both studies (Foster et al., 2010; Kowaleski-Jones and Duncan, 2002) reported what Joyce said were implausibly large improvements in outcome for the WIC mothers—a 6.6 percentage point decrease in low-birth-weight births in the first, and a 9 percentage point decrease in the second.

Propensity Score Matching

Propensity score matching has become popular in studies of WIC, but Joyce said it is more suited for use as a diagnostic. That is, propensity score matching can be used to check on the suitability of non-participants as a comparison group. The matching technique is more likely to be useful if the

WIC participants and non-participants have similar propensity scores (i.e., scores that reflect the probability of participating in WIC).

Methods for Improving Studies

Joyce said that it is important to conduct some randomized design studies because they control variation in the intervention and they are useful for testing the observational methods. That is, they provide information on how well regression, propensity score matching, and instrumental variables control for unobservable variables. He suggested that the research agenda include a small number of randomized studies of augmented care (called *WIC Plus* by earlier presenters). In addition, researchers could exploit natural sources of exogenous variation, such as twinning (if naturally occurring) and changes that provide sharp, transparent breaks in the availability of WIC services (e.g., the end of infant formula feeding at age 1 year, incidents that cause extensive damage to WIC offices and cause their closure, or variation in the timing of the rollout of a programmatic change). Regression discontinuity designs also can be helpful. Joyce encouraged researchers to think creatively, saying that WIC is paying women not to breastfeed and asking why it wouldn't be possible to pay them *to* breastfeed.

Conclusions

Joyce concluded by saying that all studies are biased until proven otherwise, sources of variation must be transparent, causal pathways need to be elucidated, and outcomes will change slowly because behavior changes slowly. A long-term research agenda would likely improve WIC research.

OPEN DISCUSSION

Moderator: Gail G. Harrison

The open discussion focused primarily on methodological issues. Participants made new or clarifying points that included the following:

- The more that dietary intakes vary from day to day, the larger the subsample should be of people providing 2-day diet recalls, and there may be some value to obtaining information on a third day's intake.
- The end of a certification period may provide a useful break in receipt of services.
- Qualitative research is helpful in explaining why models fail or why research methods are producing erroneous answers, but, Joyce said, it does not provide information about causality.

- Fixed methods control only for time-invariant factors.
- In WIC, cluster-randomized trials would involve the random assignment of clinics to treatments. The outcomes are measured at the individual level. Cluster-randomized trials ordinarily require much larger samples than do individually randomized trials. However, it appears that the sample size requirements for cluster-randomized trials of dietary intake are somewhat smaller than the requirements for studies of other outcomes.
- A better synthesis is needed of biology, sociology, and research methods. What is implausible to the methodologist may be completely plausible to a biologist and pediatrician, for example.

CLOSING REMARKS

Presenter: Gail G. Harrison

Harrison highlighted the following key research topics that were identified during the workshop sessions:

- Effects of the revised WIC food package on diet and many other behaviors. The uneven rollout of the change affords good research opportunities.
- Long-term effects of WIC on both maternal and child health, e.g., WIC plus 5 years, WIC plus 10 years, and the child upon reaching 21 years.
- The economic context for families and the implications for food security.

Regarding methods, Harrison emphasized the importance of selecting appropriate outcomes, the need to consider possible biases and timing issues, the potential value of the phased approach described by Whitaker and Taveras, the value of the applying the logic model described by Findley, and the need to rely on multiple studies with multiple methods, as indicated by Gleason and Joyce. Over the course of the workshop, participants called for both programmatic and research partnering, and the National Children's Study was mentioned many times as a possible resource with which to address some of the long-term research topics.

At Harrison's invitation, Jay Hirschman made a final statement and once again encouraged all present to send their recommendations for the top three research priorities to the Institute of Medicine website within the next few days so that the recommendations could be considered by the U.S. Department of Agriculture within its tight timeline.

REFERENCES

El-Bastawissi, A. Y., R. Peters, K. Sasseen, T. Bell, and R. Manolopoulos. 2007. Effect of the Washington Special Supplemental Nutrition Program for Women, Infants, and Children (WIC) on pregnancy outcomes. *Maternal and Child Health Journal* 11(6):611–621.

Figlio, D., S. Hamersma, and J. Roth. 2009. Does prenatal WIC participation improve birth outcomes? New evidence from Florida. *Journal of Public Economics* 93(1-2):235–245.

Foster, E. M., M. Jiang, and C. M. Gibson-Davis. 2010. The effect of the WIC program on the health of newborns. *Health Services Research* 45(4):1083–1104.

Gueorguieva, R., S. B. Morse, and J. Roth. 2009. Length of prenatal participation in WIC and risk of delivering a small for gestational age infant: Florida, 1996–2004. *Maternal and Child Health Journal* 13(4):479–488.

Kowaleski-Jones, L., and G. J. Duncan. 2002. Effects of participation in the WIC program on birthweight: Evidence from the national longitudinal survey of youth. Special Supplemental Nutrition Program for Women, Infants, and Children. *American Journal of Public Health* 92(5):799–804.

A

Workshop Agenda

HEALTH IMPACTS OF WIC—PLANNING A RESEARCH AGENDA
July 20–21, 2010, Workshop Agenda

St. Gregory Luxury Hotel & Suites, St. Gregory Ballroom
2033 M Street, NW
Washington, DC 20036

Tuesday, July 20, 2010: Day 1

Opening Session

8:00 a.m. — Welcome, Introductions, and Purpose
Gail Harrison, University of California, Los Angeles, Workshop Planning Committee Chair

Perspectives from USDA
Jay Hirschman, Special Nutrition Staff, Food and Nutrition Service

Perspectives from National WIC Association
Reverend Douglas Greenaway, President and CEO

Opening Remarks
David Paige, Johns Hopkins Bloomberg School of Public Health

Session 1: WIC and Birth Outcomes

8:30	Moderator:	*Gail Harrison, Chair*
	Speakers:	*Michael Lu, University of California, Los Angeles* *Theodore Joyce, City University of New York*
	Discussants:	*Marianne Bitler, University of California, Irvine* *Patrick Catalano, Case Western Reserve*
9:45	Break	

Session 2: WIC and Overweight and Obesity

10:05	Moderator:	*Patricia Crawford, University of California, Berkeley*
	Speakers:	*Robert Whitaker, Temple University* *Elsie Taveras, Harvard Medical School (via teleconference)*
	Discussant:	*Sara Benjamin Neelon, Duke University Medical Center*

Session 3: WIC and Breastfeeding

11:05	Moderator:	*Miriam Labbok, University of North Carolina, Chapel Hill*
	Speakers:	*Karen Bonuck, Albert Einstein College of Medicine* *Maya Bunik, University of Colorado, Children's Hospital, Denver* *Cynthia Howard, University of Rochester, School of Medicine*
	Discussant:	*Larry Grummer-Strawn, Centers for Disease Control and Prevention*
12:20 p.m.	Lunch	

Session 4: Food Insecurity and Hunger

1:30 Moderator: *Maureen Black, University of Maryland, School of Medicine*

Speakers: *John Cook, Boston Medical Center*
Edward Frongillo, University of South Carolina

Discussant: *James Weill, Food Research and Action Center*

Session 5: Dietary Intake and Nutritional Status

2:30 Moderator: *Barbara Devaney, Mathematica Policy Research*

Speakers: *Nancy Cole, Mathematica Policy Research*
Nancy Krebs, University of Colorado, Denver

Discussant: *Suzanne Murphy, University of Hawaii*

3:30 Break

Session 6: Nutrition Education

3:50 Moderator: *Shannon Whaley, PHFE–WIC Program*

Speakers: *Lorrene Ritchie, University of California, Berkeley*
Marilyn Townsend, University of California, Davis

Discussants: *Maureen Black, University of Maryland, School of Medicine*
Loren Bell, Altarum Institute

5:05 Discussion Period

5:30 Adjourn

Wednesday, July 21, 2010: Day 2

Session 7: Health Care and Systems Costs, Benefits, and Effectiveness

8:00 a.m.	Moderator:	*Barbara Devaney, Mathematica Policy Research*
	Speakers:	*Sally Findley, Columbia University* *Helen Jensen, Iowa State University*
	Discussant:	*Paul Buescher, University of North Carolina*

Session 8: The Reach of WIC

9:00	Moderator:	*Jackson Sekhobo, New York State Department of Health*
	Speakers:	*Susan Bartlett, ABT Associates* *Loren Bell, Altarum Institute*
	Discussant:	*Zoë Neuberger, Center on Budget and Policy Priorities*
10:00		Break

Closing Session: Wrap-Up and Methodological Issues and Data Considerations

10:20	Highlights of Previous Sessions *Moderators*	
11:20	Methodological Issues and Data Considerations Moderator:	*Gail Harrison, Chair*
	Speakers:	*Philip Gleason, Mathematica Policy Research* *Theodore Joyce, City University of New York*
12:20 p.m.	Open Discussion (including comments from participants)	
12:45	Summary of Key Elements of the Workshop *Gail Harrison, Chair*	

B

Biographical Sketches of the Presenters

Susan Bartlett, Ph.D., is currently a Principal Associate at Abt Associates in Cambridge, MA. For the past 25 years she has been involved in policy research primarily focused on issues concerning food and nutrition assistance programs, including WIC, the Supplemental Nutrition Assistance Program (SNAP), and the U.S. Department of Agriculture's (USDA's) school meals programs. She is currently involved in several evaluation projects to assess the impact of fruit and vegetable interventions. Dr. Bartlett holds a Ph.D. in urban and regional studies from the Massachusetts Institute of Technology.

Loren Bell, B.A., is a Subject Matter Expert at Altarum Institute and is a nationally known expert in food assistance and nutrition education program policy and program operations. He has more than 25 years' experience working with WIC and SNAP at the state and national levels. Mr. Bell has managed a number of projects, including two studies examining the food purchasing patterns of WIC clients, four food stamp nutrition education technical assistance and evaluation projects, two national studies of WIC vendor management practices, and a needs assessment of adolescents participating in the WIC program. In addition, Mr. Bell has managed a number of technical assistance efforts, including projects to help states revise how local WIC agencies are funded; conducting assessments for states developing participant-centered nutrition education in their WIC programs; and assisting states with using program data for improved program management. Mr. Bell has also directed an effort for USDA to examine the links among obesity, poverty, and participation in food assistance programs. For 11 years, Mr. Bell directed the Washington state WIC program. Mr. Bell holds a bachelor's degree in communications and undertook graduate studies in business and organizational communications at California State University, Fullerton.

Sara Benjamin Neelon, Ph.D., M.P.H., R.D., is Assistant Professor in the Department of Community and Family Medicine at Duke University Medical Center and the Duke Global Health Institute. Prior to going to Duke, Dr. Benjamin Neelon was a postdoctoral research fellow for the Obesity Prevention Program in the Department of Population Medicine at Harvard Medical School. Her research focuses on nutrition and physical activity interventions for children from birth to 5 years of age; the nutrition and physical activity environment in child care settings; early childhood predictors of obesity; feeding practices as predictors of later obesity; and nutrition policy and regulation in child care. She has published a book on nutrition for children in child care: *Making Food Healthy and Safe for Children: How to Meet the National Health and Safety Performance Standards—Guidelines for Out-of-Home Child Care Programs and Nutrition and Physical Activity in Child Care.* Dr. Benjamin Neelon received both her M.P.H. and Ph.D. in nutrition from the University of North Carolina, Chapel Hill.

Marianne P. Bitler, Ph.D., is an Associate Professor of Economics at the University of California, Irvine and a Faculty Research Associate at the National Bureau of Economic Research, Children's Program and Health Economics Program. She is also an economist at the San Francisco Federal Reserve Bank. Her research interests include labor economics, health economics, public economics, and applied microeconomics. Dr. Bitler has published in numerous economics and medical journals, including several articles on WIC, which appeared in the *Journal of Human Resources,* the *Journal of Policy Analysis and Management,* and the *Review of Agricultural Economics.* Dr. Bitler is also a member of a National Academy of Sciences Committee on Estimating Children Eligible for School Nutrition Programs Using the American Community Survey. She has a Ph.D. in economics from the Massachusetts Institute of Technology.

Maureen Black, Ph.D., M.A., is the John A. Scholl M.D. and Mary Louise Scholl M.D. Professor of Pediatrics at the University of Maryland School of Medicine and Director of the Growth and Nutrition Clinic, a multidisciplinary clinic for children with poor growth and feeding problems. She is an adjunct professor in the Center for Human Nutrition, Johns Hopkins Bloomberg School of Public Health and in the Department of Psychology, University of Maryland Baltimore County. Dr. Black is a pediatric psychologist; she has been the president of the Society of Pediatric Psychology and the Division of Children, Youth, and Family Services of the American Psychological Association. She specializes in intervention research related to children's nutrition, health, and development. She is a site principal investigator for Children's Health Watch and is conducting three National Institute Health–funded intervention trials. She is Chair of the Child Health Foundation, Vice Chair of the Maryland WIC Advisory Committee, and has served on committees for UNICEF, the World Health Organization (WHO), and the Institute of Medicine (IOM). Dr. Black has conducted four studies related to WIC: a statewide survey of feeding practices among families of infants receiving WIC, a statewide study of food preferences related to changes in the WIC food package, a study demonstrating that infants who receive WIC achieve healthier weight and lengths and are perceived to be in better health than eligible infants who do not receive WIC, and a randomized controlled trial of health promotion/obesity prevention among WIC-enrolled mothers of toddlers. She received her Ph.D. from Emory University.

Karen Bonuck, Ph.D., is an Associate Professor in the Department of Family and Social Medicine and the Department of Obstetrics, Gynecology and Women's Health at Albert Einstein College of Medicine. Her research focuses on infant and young child feeding, growth, and development. She heads two National Institutes of Health (NIH) randomized controlled trials of breastfeeding promotion interventions in low-income, multi-ethnic Bronx women. These trials, which completed enrollment of nearly 1,000 women in July 2010, are examining the effects of having an International Board Certified Lactation Consultant as part of the prenatal health care team, as well as the effects of electronically prompted prenatal care provider encouragement to breastfeed. The trials include the collection of qualitative data from both participants and providers. A secondary outcome being examined is the effect of breastfeeding on infant illnesses. Being interested in subjects across the continuum of infant feeding, Dr. Bonuck also works on the pernicious effects of extended bottle use in WIC toddlers as the principal investigator of a National Institute of Food and Agriculture randomized controlled trial and observational study.

Paul A. Buescher, Ph.D., is Adjunct Professor in the Department of Maternal and Child Health of the University of North Carolina (UNC) and a Research Fellow with the Cecil G. Sheps Center for Health Services Research at UNC. He is also a consultant to the Cancer Surveillance Branch of the U.S. Centers for Disease Control and Prevention (CDC). Dr. Buescher is retired from 32 years of state government service in North Carolina. As director of the State Center for Health Statistics in North Carolina, he was responsible for overseeing the Health and Spatial Analysis Unit, the Central Cancer Registry, the Birth Defects Monitoring Program, the Statistical Services Unit, and the Operations Unit. In several roles over 29 years at the State Center, he participated in and published many studies, especially ones related to maternal and child health. He served as project director for the CDC Pregnancy Risk Assessment Monitoring System (PRAMS) and the Behavioral Risk Factor Surveillance System (BRFSS) in North Carolina. He received his Ph.D. in sociology and demography from the University of North Carolina at Chapel Hill.

Maya Bunik, M.D., M.S.P.H., F.A.B.M., F.A.A.P., is Associate Professor of Pediatrics at the University of Colorado at Denver. She is also medical director of the primary care clinic at the Children's Hospital. As a pediatrician, she has been helping low-income mothers and babies with breastfeeding for more than 15 years. Dr. Bunik currently sees premature and other high-risk infants as part of her faculty breastfeeding practice. She has published on breastfeeding topics that concern low-income Latinas, especially the issue of "los dos" combination feeding as well as breastfeeding curriculum development for residents. Dr. Bunik received her M.D. from the University of Minnesota, Twin Cities Medical School.

Patrick M. Catalano, M.D., F.A.C.O.G., is Professor and Chair of the Department of Reproductive Biology at Case Western Reserve University at MetroHealth Medical Center. Dr. Catalano also serves on the Management Council and Executive Committee at MetroHealth Medical Center as well as on the editorial board of the *American Journal of Physiology*. He has published more than 130 articles in peer-reviewed journals and served on the editorial boards of the *Journal of Clinical Endocrinology* and *Metabolism and Diabetes*. He holds membership in the American College of Obstetricians and Gynecologists, the American Diabetes Association, the Perinatal Research Society, and the American Gynecological and Obstetrical Society. Dr. Catalano is a member of the Maternal–Fetal Medicine Division of the American Board of Obstetrics and Gynecology. Dr. Catalano's research focus is insulin resistance and glucose metabolism in pregnancy and the role of placental cytokines in the regulation of fetal growth and adiposity. He has had research support from the National Institute of Child Health and Human Development (NICHD) for more than 20 years. Dr. Catalano received his M.D. from the University of Vermont, Burlington. He served his internship at the University of California, San Francisco, and residency and postdoctoral fellowship at the University of Vermont, Burlington. Dr. Catalano is certified by the American Board of Obstetrics and Gynecology in maternal and fetal medicine.

Nancy Cole, Ph.D., is a Senior Researcher at Mathematica Policy Research, Inc. She has 17 years of experience in program evaluation for the U.S. Department of Agriculture. Dr. Cole has conducted studies of the nation's major nutrition assistance programs—food stamps (now the Supplemental Nutrition Assistance Program), WIC, the National School Lunch Program, and the Child and Adult Care Food Program. Her areas of expertise include eligibility determinations, food stamp benefit redemption patterns, computer matching and record linkage, and nutrition research. Her work has been published in the *Journal of Human Resources*. Dr. Cole obtained her Ph.D. in economics from the University of California, Los Angeles

John Cook, Ph.D., M.A.Ed., is one of the principal investigators for Children's HealthWatch, a multi-site pediatric research center based at Boston Medical Center. His research interests include examining the effects of hunger, food insecurity, and energy insecurity on child and maternal health and well-being and ways to increase access to affordable, healthful food. Research in progress is related to effects of food insecurity at its lowest levels of severity, including "marginal food security." Prior to joining Children's HealthWatch, Dr. Cook was a faculty member at Tufts University School of Nutrition Science and Policy. He is currently an Associate Professor in the Department of Pediatrics at Boston University School of Medicine. Dr. Cook received his B.A. from the University of Alabama in mathematics and Spanish and his M.A.Ed. from Arizona State University in educational psychology. He received his Ph.D. from the University of North Carolina at Chapel Hill in planning for developing areas with concentrations in demography and economics.

Patricia Crawford, Dr.P.H., R.D., is Co-Director of the Center for Weight and Health, Cooperative Extension Nutrition Specialist in the Department of Nutritional Sciences and Adjunct Professor in the School of Public Health and Department of Nutritional Sciences and Toxicology at the University of California, Berkeley. Dr. Crawford directed the 10-year longitudinal the National Heart, Lung, and Blood Institute (NHLBI) Growth & Health Study, a study of the development of cardiovascular risk factors in African American and White girls, as well as the Five-State FitWIC Initiative to Prevent Pediatric Overweight. She has developed numerous obesity-prevention materials, including the Fit Families novella series for Latino families and Let's Getting Moving, an activity program for those who work with young children. Dr. Crawford's current studies include evaluations of large community-based obesity initiatives and school-based policy interventions. Dr. Crawford is a member of the IOM standing Committee on Childhood Obesity Prevention and chaired the planning committee for a series of workshops on community perspectives to prevent childhood obesity. She earned a B.S. from the University of Washington and a Dr.P.H. and an R.D. from the University of California, Berkeley.

Barbara Devaney, Ph.D., is Director of the Human Services Research Division at Mathematica Policy Research, Inc. and a nationally recognized expert in maternal and child health, nutrition, and risk-reduction programs for youth. She has played a leading role in many of Mathematica's studies of family formation, children's nutrition, and public health programs. She is co-director of Mathematica's Building Strong Families. She also oversaw Mathematica's 2002 Feeding Infants and Toddlers Study, which provided detailed information on the food and nutrient intakes of U.S. infants and toddlers. Other evaluations in which she has played a key role have focused on the school lunch and breakfast programs, WIC, and the Food Stamp Program. She was previously an Assistant Professor at Duke University and the Johns Hopkins University. Dr. Devaney has served on the IOM Subcommittee on Uses and Interpretation of Dietary Reference Intakes and the Committee to Revise the WIC Food Packages, among others. She publishes widely in peer-reviewed journals, including the *Journal of Policy Analysis and Management, American Journal of Clinical Nutrition, Journal of the American Dietetic Association*, and the *American Journal of Public Health*. She has a Ph.D. in economics from the University of Michigan.

Sally Findley, Ph.D., is a demographer-sociologist whose work is dedicated to finding creative strategies to expand opportunities for disadvantaged mothers and their children to adopt improved health promotion practices or increase adherence to recommended treatment programs. In her research, she has focused primarily on children under age 5 and has developed strategies for including health promotion activities into or alongside WIC, Head Start, Healthy Families, and other early childhood parenting programs. Growing out of this work has been an increased appreciation for the role of community health workers (CHWs), and much of her research now focuses on documenting the contributions of community health workers and developing a sustainable funding process for CHWs in New York State. She has worked through community partnerships in Northern Manhattan (New York City) to raise childhood immunization rates, improve asthma management, reduce early childhood caries, and prevent early childhood obesity. She is currently leading a Robert Wood Johnson Foundation–funded multi-year, multi-method assessment of the impact of the recent changes in the WIC food package and related counseling procedures for the state of New York.

Edward A. Frongillo, Jr., Ph.D., is Professor and Chair of the Department of Health Promotion, Education, and Behavior in the Arnold School of Public Health at the University of South Carolina in Columbia. Dr. Frongillo studies how to solve under- and over-nutrition of populations globally, especially children and families living in poverty, using qualitative and quantitative methods. His particular research interests are growth, development, and feeding of infants and young children and the role of family stress and parenting in these; measurement and consequences of household food insecurity and hunger; policies and programs for improving nutrition and development; advancement of consensus, commitment, and capacity for nutrition and health in poor locations; and design and analysis of longitudinal studies.

Philip M. Gleason, Ph.D., a Senior Fellow at Mathematica Policy Research, is an expert in evaluation design and random assignment. He has directed many studies related to education initiatives and federal nutrition programs. Dr. Gleason recently completed a rigorous evaluation of charter schools for the U.S. Department of Education and directs an evaluation of KIPP (Knowledge is Power Program) middle schools for the KIPP Foundation as well as an evaluation of Teacher Residency Programs. He recently led a study of childhood obesity and school meal programs. He has played a key role in research examining administrative and nutrition-related aspects of the school meal programs, examined the dynamics of participation in the Food Stamp Program, and studied dropout-prevention programs. Dr. Gleason publishes regularly in peer-reviewed journals, with recent articles appearing in the *Journal of Policy Analysis and Management, Evaluation Review, Journal of the American Dietetic Association, Journal of Agricultural Economics*, and *Demography.* He is also on the board of editors of the *Journal of the American Dietetic Association* and authored a chapter in *Race, Poverty, and Domestic Policy*, a book from Yale University Press. He holds a Ph.D. in economics from the University of Wisconsin, Madison.

Rev. Douglas A. Greenaway is President and Chief Executive Officer of the National WIC Association (NWA). For 20 years he has been responsible for directing the NWA as well as representing the interests of its members (50 states, 40 Indian nations, and trust territories, 2,200 local agencies, and 10,000 clinics that operate the Special Supplemental Nutrition Program for WIC) before Congress, the USDA, other federal agencies, and the White House. Fr. Greenaway was Ordained to the Holy Order of Priests in the Anglican/Episcopal Diocese of Washington and serves as Priest Associate at St. Paul's Rock Creek Parish, as Honorary Assistant at St. Paul's K Street Parish, and as on-call chaplain at Washington Hospital Center. He began work in 1974 with the Research Office of the Official Opposition in Canadian Parliament, writing speeches and debate notes for the Leader of the Official Opposition and Opposition Members of Parliament. He holds a master of divinity degree from Wesley Theological Seminary and a master of architecture degree from The Catholic University of America.

Laurence Grummer-Strawn, M.P.A., M.A., Ph.D., is Chief of the Nutrition Branch at CDC. As branch chief, he is responsible for national surveillance of nutrition among low-income children, national breastfeeding support efforts, fruit and vegetable promotion, and international micronutrient deficiency programs. He has worked at CDC for almost 19 years, in the areas of reproductive health and nutrition. He has more than 100 scientific publications. Dr. Grummer-Strawn is recognized internationally for his work on vitamin and mineral deficiencies, breastfeeding policy, and development of both the CDC and the WHO Growth Charts. He is widely known in the breastfeeding research and advocacy communities, serving as scientific editor of the Surgeon General's Call to Action on Breastfeeding, an executive committee member of the International Society for Research on Human Milk and Lactation, and a liaison to the U.S. Breastfeeding Committee. He earned his Ph.D. from Princeton University.

Gail Harrison, Ph.D., is Professor in the Department of Community Health Sciences at the University of California, Los Angeles (UCLA) School of Public Health and senior research scientist at the UCLA Center for Health and Policy Research. Previously, she was Professor in the Department of Family and Community Medicine at the University of Arizona. Dr. Harrison has worked extensively in the area of dietary and nutritional assessment of diverse populations. She is a former member of the Food and Nutrition Board and has served on several of its committees, including the Committee on International Nutrition Programs, the Committee to Review the Risk Criteria for the Women, Infants, and Children (WIC) Program, the Committee on Implications of Dioxin in the Food Supply, the Committee to Revise the WIC Food Packages, and the Committee on Nutrition Standards for National School Lunch and Breakfast Programs. She has served in various advisory capacities for the National Institutes of Health and the USDA, consulted with the World Health Organization and UNICEF, and has worked in Egypt, the Sudan, Iran, Indonesia, and Lesotho, besides the United States. Dr. Harrison has an M.N.S. (nutritional sciences) from Cornell University and a Ph.D. in physical anthropology from the University of Arizona. She also serves on the Board of the California Food Policy Advocates organization. Dr. Harrison is a Fellow of the American Society for Nutrition and a member of IOM.

Jay Hirschman, M.P.H., C.N.S., Director of the Special Nutrition Staff at the USDA Food and Nutrition Service (FNS) Office of Research and Analysis, has worked in public health nutrition at the local, state, and federal level, including 25 years at USDA/FNS. He served as a state WIC Supervisor and as the first Director for the Nutrition Policy and Analysis Staff at the then newly formed USDA Center for Nutrition Policy and Promotion.

In his current position of staff director, he is responsible for managing the staff conducting the evaluation studies and policy analysis for all domestic Special Nutrition Programs, including WIC, the National School Lunch Program (NSLP), the School Breakfast Program (SBP), the Child and Adult Care Food Program (CACFP) and the other child nutrition programs, and the Food Distribution Programs. Mr. Hirschman is an American College of Nutrition (ACN) board-certified nutrition specialist (CNS) and served as elected Chair of the American Public Health Association Food and Nutrition Section (APHA/FN) in 2003–2004. In 2009 he received the APHA/FN Mary C. Egan award, which "goes to those public health nutritionists who pioneer fresh approaches to public health nutrition, nutrition education, and those groups with special dietary needs."

Cynthia Howard, M.D., M.P.H., is Associate Professor in the Departments of Pediatrics and Community and Preventive Medicine at the University of Rochester School of Medicine and Dentistry and Pediatric Director of the Mother-Baby Unit at Rochester General Hospital. Dr. Howard focuses the majority of her research on infant nutrition, breastfeeding, and human lactation. In 2000 she lead the team that helped Rochester General Hospital become designated as a Baby Friendly hospital. She is a member of the board of directors for the New York State breastfeeding coalition, the health advisory board of La Leche League International, and the editorial board of *Birth*. She is the past President of the Academy of Breastfeeding Medicine, Co-Chairperson of the protocol committee, and the Senior Associate Editor for the journal *Breastfeeding Medicine*. Dr. Howard has served as principal investigator in several research studies on clinical breastfeeding issues and has authored many research papers and book chapters. She is a member of the Society for Pediatric Research and the International Society for Research in Human Milk and Lactation. Her current research includes a clinical study designed to evaluate vitamin D nutrition during lactation that is focusing on optimizing health outcomes for mothers and their infants. Additionally, she is an investigator on a community-based project funded by the National Institutes of Health focusing on improving breastfeeding initiation and duration in the greater Rochester area through community partnerships.

Helen H. Jensen, Ph.D., is Professor in the Department of Economics, College of Agriculture and Life Sciences at Iowa State University (ISU) and serves as head of the Food and Nutrition Policy Division in the Center for Agricultural and Rural Development (CARD) at ISU. Dr. Jensen's research concerns food demand and consumption, food assistance and nutrition policies, food security, and the economics of food safety and hazard control. She has been a member of the board of directors of the American Agricultural Economics Association and serves on the editorial board of a number of professional journals. Dr. Jensen was a member of the IOM Committee on Nutrition Standards for National School Lunch and Breakfast Programs and on the IOM Committee to Review the WIC Food Packages. She also served on the National Research Council (NRC) Committee on National Statistics panel to review USDA's measurement of food insecurity and hunger and on other NRC committees related to the U.S. sheep industry and animal health and diseases. She is currently a member of the IOM Committee to Review CACFP Meal Requirements and the NRC Committee on Ranking FDA Product Categories Based on Health Consequences. Dr. Jensen holds a B.A. in economics from Carleton College, an M.S. in agricultural and applied economics from the University of Minnesota, and a Ph.D. in agricultural economics from the University of Wisconsin, Madison.

Theodore Joyce, Ph.D., is a National Bureau of Economics Research Associate in the Programs on Health Economics and Children and a Professor of Economics at Baruch College and the Graduate Center of the City University of New York. He is also the Academic Director of the Baruch/Mount Sinai MBA Program in Health Care Administration, in which he teaches health economics and statistics. Dr. Joyce received his B.A. in bilingual education from the University of Massachusetts in 1976 and his Ph.D. in economics from the City University of New York in 1985. Professor Joyce's research interests are in infant and reproductive health policy. His published work has appeared in economic, policy, and clinical journals. He is best known for his work on abortion policies and their impact on fertility and infant health.

Nancy F. Krebs, M.D., M.S., is a Professor of Pediatrics in the Department of Pediatrics at the University of Colorado Denver (UCD), and is the head of the Section of Nutrition in the Department of Pediatrics. She is board certified in general pediatrics, clinical nutrition, and pediatric gastroenterology. Dr. Krebs has extensive research experience in trace mineral nutrition in breastfeeding infants and their mothers, including in international settings. Current research in the United States is testing effects of different complementary feeding regimens to meet micronutrient requirements for breastfed infants. Through the NIH/NICHD Global Network for Women's and Children's Research, she leads an ongoing multi-country efficacy trial of complementary feeding and growth and development. As a secondary area of research interest, she is a co-investigator in research related to childhood obesity, both prevention and treatment studies. Dr. Krebs' clinical activities include directing two pediatric nutrition clinics, including one for children with undernutrition and feeding problems, and the other for overweight infants and children. She has more than 160 research and scholarly publications. She served as the Chair of the Committee on Nutrition for the American Academy of Pediatrics for 4 years, and as Co-Chair of the AAP Task Force on Obesity. From 2003–2007, she served as a member of the Food and Nutrition Board with the National Academy of Sciences. Dr. Krebs earned her M.D. from UCD School of Medicine.

Miriam H. Labbok, M.D., M.P.H., M.M.S., F.A.C.P.M., F.A.B.M., I.B.C.L.C., has been Professor of the Practice of Public Health, and Director, Carolina Global Breastfeeding Institute (CGBI) since January 2006. Previously, Dr. Labbok served as the Senior Advisor for infant and young child feeding and care at UNICEF headquarters; Chief, Maternal Health and Nutrition Division, Global Health Bureau, and Medical Officer, Population Bureau, U.S. Agency for International Development (USAID); Associate Professor at Georgetown University Medical Center, Director of the WHO Center of Excellence on Breastfeeding, and Co-Director, Institute for Reproductive Health; Assistant Professor, Johns Hopkins School of Hygiene and Public Health, and Adjunct Associate Professor at Tulane. She is a graduate of University of Pennsylvania with general honors; the University of Medicine and Dentistry of New Jersey–Rutgers; and Tulane University (where she studied under the mentorship of Dr. Cicely Williams). She was a resident in pediatrics at Georgetown University Medical Center and completed post-doctoral research in epidemiology with honors and a preventive medicine residency at Johns Hopkins. Dr. Labbok has 35 years of research, technical assistance, training, and program development experience related to maternal/child dyad health and nutrition issues. She has worked in more than 50 countries and is known for her contributions to the development and testing of the lactational amenorrhea method (LAM) for family planning. She has been very involved in a birth spacing/family planning program and policy for health outcomes. Recently, her research on breastfeeding has focused primarily on disparities, and workplace-, hospital-, and community-based health initiatives using operational and translational epidemiological approaches. As a result of her work on breastfeeding, LAM, family planning, and the reproductive health continuum, she has been recognized with honors as varied as distinguished alumnus of all institutions of higher learning attended, the first Science and Technology Award from USAID, both student and distinguished honoree of La Leche League International (LLLI), faculty Delta Omega, and many others. She has published more than 300 chapters, articles, monographs, and abstracts, and she has presented hundreds of invited lectures and seminars.

Michael C. Lu, M.D., M.P.H., M.S., is an Associate Professor of Obstetrics & Gynecology and Public Health at the University of California, Los Angeles (UCLA) School of Medicine. His research focuses on racial/ethnic disparities in birth outcomes from a life-course perspective. Dr. Lu is widely recognized for his research, teaching, and clinical care. He received the 2003 National Maternal and Child Health Epidemiology Young Professional Award and the 2004 American Public Health Association Maternal and Child Health Young Professional Award for his research on health disparities. Dr. Lu has previously served on several IOM committees, including the Committee on Understanding Premature Birth and Assuring Health Outcomes, and the Committee to Reexamine Pregnancy Weight Guidelines. He has also received numerous awards for his teaching, including Excellence in Teaching awards from the Association of Professors of Gynecology and Obstetrics. Dr. Lu maintains an active clinical practice in obstetrics and gynecology at UCLA Medical Center and has been selected as one of the Best Doctors in America since 2005. Dr. Lu received a B.A. in human biology and political science from Stanford University, an M.S. in health and medical sciences, an M.P.H. in epidemiology from the University of California, Berkeley, and an M.D. from the University of California, San Francisco School of Medicine.

Suzanne P. Murphy, Ph.D., R.D., is a Researcher and Professor at the Cancer Research Center of Hawaii at the University of Hawaii and Director of the Nutrition Support Shared Resource at the center. Dr. Murphy's research interests include dietary assessment methodology, development of food composition databases, and nutritional epidemiology of chronic diseases (with an emphasis on cancer and obesity). Dr. Murphy has served as a member of the National Nutrition Monitoring Advisory Council and the year 2000 Dietary Guidelines Advisory Committee. She is a member of various professional organizations, including the American Dietetic Association, the American Society for Nutrition, the American Public Health Association, the Society for Nutrition Education, and the Society for Epidemiological Research. Dr. Murphy has served on several IOM committees. She chaired the Subcommittee on Interpretation and Uses of Dietary Reference Intakes and the Committee to Review the WIC Food Packages, was a member of the Committee to Review the National School Lunch and School Breakfast Programs, and currently chairs the Committee to Review the Child and Adult Care Food Program Meal Requirements. She is also a member of the Food and Nutrition Board. Dr. Murphy earned an M.S. in molecular biology from San Francisco State University and a Ph.D. in nutrition from the University of California, Berkeley. She is a registered dietitian.

Zoë Neuberger, J.D., is a Senior Policy Analyst at the Center on Budget and Policy Priorities, where she has worked since 2001. She primarily works on the school meal programs and WIC, providing analytic and technical assistance to policymakers and state-level nonprofit groups. Previously, she worked as an analyst at the White House Office of Management and Budget, where she was responsible for oversight of federal spending on Temporary Assistance for Needy Families, child care, child nutrition, WIC, and low-income tax credits. She holds a law degree from Yale University and a master in public policy degree from Harvard's Kennedy School of Government.

David Paige, M.D., M.P.H., is Professor of Population and Family Health with a joint appointment in International Health and Human Nutrition at the Johns Hopkins Bloomberg School of Public Health and a joint appointment in Pediatrics at the School of Medicine. He is an expert in the area of community health and maternal and child nutrition. Dr. Paige's groundbreaking studies of lactose intolerance in children, his pioneering effort in establishing a supplemental feeding program for disadvantaged women, infants, and children, and his design and implementation of community-based programs define the scope of his interest. His design and implementation of a supplemental feeding program served as the prototype for the USDA Supplemental Nutrition Program for Women, Infants, and Children. He is a contributor to the professional literature and is the author of numerous chapters and articles in scientific journals. Dr. Paige edited the textbook *Clinical Nutrition* and is the past Editor-in-Chief of the journal *Clinical Nutrition.* He has been a member of numerous national scientific panels and committees and has served as consultant to federal, state, and local governments, most recently having served as a reviewer for the Institute of Medicine publication on the redesign of the USDA WIC Program. He is the recipient of numerous awards, including the March of Dimes National Agnes Higgins Award for Distinguished Achievement in Maternal–Fetal Nutrition.

Lorrene Ritchie, Ph.D., R.D., is Director of Research at the Dr. Robert C. and Veronica Atkins Center for Weight and Health at the University of California, Berkeley. She has worked for more than a decade to promote the development of interdisciplinary, science-based, and culturally relevant solutions to the obesity epidemic in children and families. She served as an evidence analyst for the American Dietetic Association (ADA) and co-authored the ADA's position paper on pediatric weight management. She recently served as a member of the ADA's Pediatric Weight Management Workgroup to formulate evidence-based practice guidelines and the California Department of Education's Child Care Nutrition Standards Workgroup to improve nutrition standards for licensed child care. She is co-author of a book, *Obesity: Dietary and Developmental Influences*, and serves as the pediatric section editor of the ADA's Weight Management Dietary Practice Group newsletter. She currently manages several research projects, including: characterizing dietary patterns and timing of eating in relation to obesity in a longitudinal cohort of Black and White girls followed through adolescence; investigating the nutrition environments in childcare settings in California; assessing nutrition knowledge, attitudes, and behaviors of WIC participants in response to a nutrition education campaign and the new WIC food package changes in California; and evaluating student dietary intakes and school food environment changes related to USDA's Fresh Fruit and Vegetable Program. Dr. Ritchie obtained her doctorate in nutrition at the University of California, Berkeley.

Jackson P. Sekhobo, Ph.D., M.P.A., is Director, Evaluation and Analysis Unit, Bureau of Administration & Evaluation, Division of Nutrition with the New York State Department of Health. Previously, he was an evaluation consultant for the New York City Department of Health and Mental Hygiene for the New York City Diabetes Registry project, and an Assistant Medical Professor for the Sophie Davis School of Biomedical Education, City College of New York, City University of New York. Dr. Sekhobo is currently working on a NY Fit WIC Grant: Revitalizing WIC Nutrition Service, and he is leading the study, "First Steps" Evaluation of New York State Childhood Obesity Prevention Policies, which is being funded by the Robert Wood Johnson Foundation and the New York State Health Foundation. Dr. Sekhobo received his M.P.A. in health policy from New York University and his Ph.D. in epidemiology from the University of Albany, State University of New York.

Elsie M. Taveras, M.D., M.P.H., is Assistant Professor of both Population Medicine and Pediatrics at Harvard Medical School's Department of Population Medicine (DPM). She works with DPM's Center for Child Health Care Studies and co-directs DPM's Obesity Prevention Program. She is also the Director of the One Step Ahead clinic, a multidisciplinary childhood overweight prevention and early management program at Children's Hospital Boston. Her research interests include nutrition and physical activity as they affect child health and childhood obesity prevention. Dr. Taveras is a recipient of the Physician Faculty Scholars Program of the Robert Wood Johnson Foundation to examine opportunities for childhood obesity prevention among underserved populations. Dr. Taveras trained in pediatrics at Children's Hospital Boston and Boston Medical Center and received her M.P.H. from the Harvard School of Public Health.

Marilyn Townsend, Ph.D., R.D., is the Cooperative Extension Nutrition Specialist in the Department of Nutrition at the University of California, Davis. Dr. Townsend has extensive experience in program evaluation, having conducted randomized controlled trials and quasi-experimental evaluation studies in low-income communities. She has conducted studies on mediators of behavior change with both adult and youth audiences. Her work includes theory-driven program development and implementation, nutrition educational methodologies, and program evaluation. She is an expert on the development of assessment tools for primary prevention interventions for low-literate audiences in low-income communities. Specifically, she focuses on tools for program evaluation and risk assessment conducting studies for validation, reliability, and sensitivity to change. She is the recipient of the Sustained Excellence in Extension Evaluation Award, sponsored by the American Evaluation Association, Extension Education Evaluation Topical Interest Group, the Jeanne M. Priester Award for outstanding health education intervention, and the Dannon Institute's Award in Community Nutrition. She obtained her M.S. in nutrition science from the University of London (Kings College) and then her Ph.D. in nutrition with emphasis on behavior from Pennsylvania State University.

James Weill, J.D., has been President of the Food Research and Action Center (FRAC) since February 1998. FRAC is the leading anti-hunger public policy group in America, using research, policy advocacy, coalition building, and public education to combat hunger and improve nutrition for low-income people. He has devoted his entire professional career to reducing hunger and poverty, protecting the legal rights of children and poor people, and expanding economic security, income, and nutrition support programs and health insurance coverage. Prior to joining FRAC, he was at the Children's Defense Fund (CDF) as Program Director and General Counsel, leading CDF's efforts to expand the Earned Income Tax Credit, Medicaid, and other programs. Mr. Weill is a member of the boards of OMB Watch and the National Center for Youth Law. He serves on advisory councils to the National League of Cities Institute for Youth, Education and Families and to Wider Opportunities for Women. He has served as a member of the U.S. delegation to the UNICEF executive board. His undergraduate degree is from Cornell and his law degree is from New York University.

Shannon Whaley, Ph.D., is the Director of Research and Evaluation at Public Health Foundation Enterprise (PHFE)–WIC Program, the largest local agency WIC program in the nation. PHFE-WIC serves more than 316,000 women, infants, and children every month in Los Angeles and Orange Counties, translating into 4 percent of the nation's total WIC participants. Dr. Whaley's expertise is in the planning, development, and evaluation of programs designed to optimize the healthy development of young children and families. Her work spans a broad range of topics, including childhood nutrition, prevention of prenatal alcohol use, obesity prevention, and promotion of early literacy for low-income children, and it includes controlled research studies as well as implementation of community-based interventions using evidenced-based practices. Dr. Whaley received her B.A in psychology from Pomona College and her Ph.D. in developmental psychology from UCLA.

Robert C. Whitaker, M.D., M.P.H., is Professor of Public Health and Pediatrics at Temple University's Center for Obesity Research and Education. Prior to joining the Temple faculty, he was a Senior Fellow at Mathematica Policy Research, Inc. in Princeton, New Jersey, and a visiting Senior Research Scholar at the Center for Health and Wellbeing at the Woodrow Wilson School of Public and International Affairs at Princeton University. His research has focused on the childhood antecedents of adult chronic disease. This has included studies on school nutrition, obesity prevention strategies in preschool children, parent–child feeding interactions, the epidemiology of childhood obesity, and the determinants of social and emotional well-being in children. He served on the IOM Committee on Dietary Risk Assessment in the WIC Program and the Committee on Prevention of Obesity in Children and Youth. Dr. Whitaker received a B.A. in chemistry from Williams College, an M.D. from the Johns Hopkins University School of Medicine, and an M.P.H. from the University of Washington School of Public Health and Community Medicine. Dr. Whitaker completed his residency and fellowship in pediatrics at the University of Washington School of Medicine, and he received postdoctoral training as a Robert Wood Johnson Clinical Scholar.

C

Workshop Attendees

Joanne Arsenault
Nutrition Policy Analyst
RTI International

Michael Burke
Food Research and Action Center

Annina Burns
Study Director
Food and Nutrition Board
Institute of Medicine
The National Academies

Arianna Caroghi
Sun-Maid

Jasmine Chan
N. Chapman Associates, Inc.

Nancy Chapman
President
N. Chapman Associates, Inc.

Ann Collins
Principal Associate
Abt Associates

Kristina Davis
Prevention Science Fellow
Office of Disease Prevention and Health Promotion
U.S. Department of Health and Human Services

Laura Dotson
Nutrition Intern
Food Research and Action Center

Catherine Dunham
Executive Director
Children's Dental Health Project

Leslie Erdelack
Association of State and Territorial Health Officials

Kenneth Finegold
Program Analyst
Assistant Secretary for Planning and Evaluation
U.S. Department of Health and Human Services

Stacey Flanagan
Director, Public Health Service Programs
Public Health Solutions

Mary Kay Fox
Senior Researcher
Mathematica Policy Research, Inc.

Tracy Fox
President
Food, Nutrition & Policy Consultants, LLC

Betsy Frazao
Economic Research Service
U.S. Department of Agriculture

Denise Gee
Senior Nutritionist
Public Health Foundation Enterprises WIC Program

Judy Gomez
Director of Planning and Projects
Public Health Foundation Enterprises WIC Program

Pat Gradziel
Health Program Specialist
California WIC Program

Mary Gray
Economic Research Service
U.S. Department of Agriculture

Melanie Hall
Nutrition Marketing–WIC
Kellogg

Isadora Hare
Perinatal Health Specialist
Health Resources and Services Administration
Maternal and Child Health Bureau

Suzanne Harris
Executive Director
ILSI Research Foundation

Heather Hartline-Grafton
Senior Nutrition Policy Analyst
Food Research and Action Center

Paulette Helman
Registered Dietitian
Private Practice

Geraldine Henchy
Director of Nutrition Policy
Food Research and Action Center

Amy Hillier
Assistant Professor
University of Pennsylvania

Donna Hines
Acting Branch Chief
Food and Nutrition Service
U.S. Department of Agriculture

Judy Hirigoyen
Executive Director
California Dried Fruit Coalition

Jay Hirschman
Director, Special Nutrition Staff
Office of Research and Analysis
Food and Nutrition Service
U.S. Department of Agriculture

Nicole Holovach
Research Associate
Food and Nutrition Board
Institute of Medicine
The National Academies

Lisa Honig
Children's Dental Health Project

Eloise Jenks
Deputy Director
Public Health Foundation Enterprises WIC Program

William Kaericher
Director, Government Food Programs
Beech Nut Nutrition Corporation

Lucia Kaiser
CE Specialist
University of California, Davis

Marta Kealey
Nutritionist
Food and Nutrition Service
U.S. Department of Agriculture

Monique LaRocque
Vice President
Feinstein Kean Healthcare

Laura Leviton
Special Advisor on Evaluation
Robert Wood Johnson Foundation

Patricia MacNeal
Nutritionist
Center for Nutrition Policy and Promotion
U.S. Department of Agriculture

Katie Martin
Research Analyst
California Maternal, Child and Adolescent Health

Doris McGuire
Altarum Institute

Jackie McLaughlin
M.P.H. Program Associate Director
University of Pennsylvania

Elizabeth Metallinos-Katsaras
Associate Professor, Nutrition Department
Simmons College

Stephen Michael
Policy Directions Inc.

Patti Mitchell
Senior Program Analyst
Food and Nutrition Service
U.S. Department of Agriculture

Carolyn Mullen
March of Dimes

Beth Myers
Temple University

Vic Oliveira
Economist
Economic Research Service
U.S. Department of Agriculture

Rani Patel
Director
Native Health, WIC

Cynthia Pellegrini
Associate Director, Federal Affairs
American Academy of Pediatrics

Mary Pat Raimondi
Vice President, Strategic Policy and Partnerships
American Dietetic Association

Julie Reeder
Senior Research Analyst
Oregon WIC Program

Cecilia Richardson
Staff/Nutrition Programs Director
National WIC Association

Joseph Robare
Research Analyst
Food and Nutrition Service
U.S. Department of Agriculture

Sarah Roholt
Nutrition Program Supervisor
North Carolina Division of Public Health

Sanna Ronkainen
Office of Disease Prevention and Health Promotion
U.S. Department of Health and Human Services

Leila Saldanha
NutrIQ LLC

Kiran Saluja
Deputy Director
Public Health Foundation Enterprises WIC Program

Jennifer Savage-Williams
Associate Director
Pennsylvania State University

Julia Schneider
Director, Chronic Disease
Association of State and Territorial Health Officials

Tamara Schryver
General Mills
Bell Institute of Health and Nutrition

Karen Sell
Bureau Chief
Arizona Department of Health Services
Bureau of Nutrition and Physical Activity

Ursaline Singleton
Nutritionist
Department of Health and Human Services

David Smallwood
FANRP Director
Economic Research Service
U.S. Department of Agriculture

Lisa Southworth
Food and Nutrition Service
U.S. Department of Agriculture

Jayaram Srinivasan
Resident Physician
Office of Disease Prevention and Health

Donna Thompson
Administrator
Maricopa Department of Public Health

Laura Tiehen
Economic Research Service
U.S. Department of Agriculture

Lisa Troy
Study Director
Food and Nutrition Board
Institute of Medicine
The National Academies

Laurie True
Executive Director
California WIC Association

Lisa Watson
Watson/Mulhern

Kurtria Watson
Nutritionist
Food and Nutrition Service
U.S. Department of Agriculture

Gwendolyn West
DC Breastfeeding Coalition

Debra Whitford
Director, Supplemental Food Programs Division
Food and Nutrition Service
U.S. Department of Agriculture

Kathleen Woolf
Research and Development Manager
Arizona Department of Health Services
Bureau of Nutrition and Physical Activity

D

Abbreviations and Acronyms

BFHI	Baby Friendly Hospital Initiative
BMI	body mass index
BRAC	Bangladesh Rural Advancement Committee
CDC	Centers for Disease Control and Prevention
EBT	electronic benefit transfer
FITS	Feeding Infant and Toddlers Study
IBCLC	International Board Certified Lactation Consultant
NHANES	National Health and Nutrition Examination Survey
NWA	National WIC Association
PCP	Primary Healthcare Provider
PHC	Primary Health Care
RCT	randomized controlled trial
SCHIP	State Children's Health Insurance Program
SNAP	Supplemental Nutrition Assistance Program
SNAP-Ed	Supplemental Nutrition Assistance Program-Education
TREND	Transparent Reporting of Evaluations with Non-randomized Designs
USDA	U.S. Department of Agriculture
WHO	World Health Organization
WIC	Supplemental Nutrition Program for Women, Infants, and Children
WIC-PC	WIC Participants and Program Characteristics

E

Excerpts from Comments Received on the Institute of Medicine's Website for the Workshop to Plan a Research Agenda for WIC

The Institute of Medicine set up a website for the workshop "Health Impacts of WIC—Planning a Research Agenda" and invited interested parties to submit comments between June 11, 2010, and August 2, 2010. During the workshop, the URL for the website was shown several times, and all persons in attendance were encouraged to submit their top three research priorities and other comments. Eight comments were received, one of which was submitted jointly by two individuals from the same company and two of which were identical. Some of the comments have been shortened (to focus on the research priorities) and copy edited. The complete set of unedited comments was forwarded to the Food and Nutrition Service of the U.S. Department of Agriculture for its consideration.

TOP RESEARCH PRIORITIES

Commenters A and B

Identical but separate suggestions from Laurie Kaiser and Laurie True of the California WIC Association:

1. Dedicate a portion of the available funds to a small, innovative demonstration research grants pool administered by a research institution with strong WIC experience and expertise. The grants pool should be distributed to test and evaluate "WIC Plus" projects in partnership with state or local programs. These funds should be

leveraged by partnering with health foundations, which should be asked to match funding for important WIC research.

2. The California WIC Association strongly supports Robert Whitaker's proposal to coordinate nutrition education and communication strategies around a series of WIC interventions. California WIC has had great success using the Sesame Healthy Habits messages in a unified messaging and education intervention that is described in a *Journal of Nutrition Education and Behavior* article.
3. Pilot and evaluate WIC breastfeeding interventions, including the distribution of generically labeled formula, in order to document what works to increase the rates and duration of exclusive breastfeeding.

Commenter C

Joanne Arsenault, Nutrition Policy Analyst, RTI International:

1. Increase breastfeeding rates; identify why rates are lower among WIC participants than among income-eligible non-participants; identify what works for promotion; and implement/standardize across the program.
2. Conduct detailed dietary surveys to determine which WIC foods are actually consumed by the target individuals, and conduct longitudinal studies to determine if nutritional risk factors decrease over time on WIC because of the consumption of WIC foods.
3. Conduct longitudinal studies to determine if WIC has an impact on overall diet quality and food insecurity.

Commenters D and E

Melanie Hall, M.S., R.D., Nutrition Marketing-WIC; and Nelson Almeida, Ph.D., F.A.C.N., V.P, US/Global Nutrition, Science, Labeling & Marketing, Kellogg Company:

1. Work with the Supplemental Nutrition Assistance Program (SNAP) to evaluate a variety of nutrition education methods.
2. Find ways to study and communicate the benefits of including produce in the new food package, for both WIC participants and retailers.
3. Investigate how the WIC program (including nutrition education and food package options) influences WIC participants' purchasing habits outside of the food package. Consider a longitudinal study that compares participants' actual buying behavior before, during,

and after participation in WIC. A longitudinal pantry study in a sample of WIC households would help WIC understand:

- how participation in WIC influences the purchase of foods with a nutrition profile that is similar to that of authorized WIC foods,
- how participation in WIC influences the purchasing of non-WIC foods,
- if purchasing habits stay the same or change once the mother's certification ends, and
- the degree and type of variance between reported consumption and actual purchasing behavior (e.g., whether behaviors are unchanged in some food segments while changing in others, and by how much).

Commenter F

Betsy Frazao, Economic Research Service:

1. Expand the availability of data for WIC research

    a. *Enhance administrative data for research and evaluation* For example, a contractor might assist in determining the types of data to be collected and made available, in what format, and how it might be linked to other data. Possible linkages include those with the Pregnancy and the Pediatric Nutrition Surveillance systems, Medicaid, and vital records. The standardization of data collection procedures across states would allow national-level analysis. Such standardization might be possible by providing states with "best practices" suggestions, financial resources, and technical assistance. The maintenance of an up-to-date state WIC policy database would be essential in interpreting and understanding the findings of the research.
    b. *Enhance state and national survey data for WIC research* Possible ways to ensure the collection of relevant data on WIC participation and outcomes include (1) the development of standardized questions on WIC participation, breastfeeding, eating behaviors, and other outcomes measures; (2) the development of supplemental WIC modules to be included in state and national surveys; and (3) the funding of the supplemental WIC modules in state and national surveys. Funding sentinel sites might also be considered as a source of data for WIC research.

c. *Provide funds to increase the sample size of current surveys*, such as the National Health and Nutrition Examination Survey or the National Children's Survey, to include more WIC participants.

2. Evaluate which WIC option yields the highest return: (1) enhancing WIC package and services to a more targeted group, or (2) expanding WIC to more people (perhaps pre-conception women).
3. Develop a cost–benefit analysis justification for breastfeeding in WIC, including estimates of the costs and benefits based on different durations and intensities of breastfeeding and depending on whether the infant is fed at the breast or fed breast milk in a bottle. Consider the costs and benefits from

   a. an individual perspective (e.g., morbidity, obesity, dietary intake, and nutritional status),
   b. the WIC perspective (e.g., participation rates, food costs, and costs of breastfeeding promotion, peer counselors, lactation consultants, and breast pumps), and
   c. a national health perspective (e.g., short-term and long-run health care costs).

Commenter G

Elizabeth Metallinos-Katsaras, Associate Professor, Nutrition Department, Simmons College:

> As a prerequisite to any implementation of a research agenda, USDA needs to provide guidance and leadership to facilitate state release of individual-level WIC data that can be used to establish linkages. The three priorities for a WIC research agenda that are listed below assume that USDA can assist states to successfully develop and implement policies of collaborative data sharing, and they address the most common nutrition-related problems (overweight and obesity) that are amenable to prevention within the WIC program. The third priority addresses how best to intervene within the WIC environment to affect health-related attitudes, behaviors, and outcomes.

1. *WIC and maternal and child obesity* What is the effect of WIC participation on maternal weight status, child weight gain velocity, and status in infancy and childhood? Which predictors (e.g., breastfeeding initiation and duration, household food insecurity) are affected by WIC and may interact with WIC to affect these outcomes?

2. *The impact of the new WIC food package* What is the effect of the new WIC food package on changes in maternal health behaviors (i.e., foods purchased, breastfeeding) and child health outcomes (i.e., weight status, weight gain velocity, food intake).
3. *Effective approaches to effecting positive health-related attitude and behavior change* How effective are the current counseling strategies to inform, encourage, and support positive health-related attitudes, behaviors, and outcomes in the WIC population; and how can they be improved to be more effective in an ethnically diverse, high-risk population?

Commenter H

Jennifer McGuire, M.S., R.D., Manager, Nutrition Communication, National Fisheries Institute:

> Research: "to better understand how best to increase the consumption of seafood, the only natural source of essential omega-3s, in the diets of WIC participants for the best possible pregnancy outcomes for both mother and child."

Studies Cited in Support of This Suggestion Appear Below

Choiniere, C. B., B. Timbo, D. Street, P. Trumbo, and S. B. Fein. 2008. *Fish consumption by women of childbearing age, pregnant women and mothers of infants.* Poster presented at the International Association for Food Protection 95th Annual Meeting, Columbus, Ohio, August 3–6.

Danaei, G., E. L. Ding, D. Mozaffarian, B. Taylor, J. Rehm, C. J. Murray, and M. Ezzati. 2009. The preventable causes of death in the United States: Comparative risk assessment of dietary, lifestyle, and metabolic risk factors. *PLoS Med* 6(4):e1000058.

Golding, J., C. Steer, P. Emmett, J. M. Davis, and J. R. Hibbeln. 2009. High levels of depressive symptoms in pregnancy with low omega-3 fatty acid intake from fish. *Epidemiology* 20(4):598–603.

Koletzko, B., I. Cetin, J. Thomas Brenna, G. Alvino, J. von Berlepsch, H. K. Biesalski, T. Clandinin, H. Debertin, T. Decsi, H. Demmelmair, G. Desoye, V. Dietz, P. Dodds, P. Emmett, F. Facchinetti, M. W. Gillman, J. Heinrich, E. Herrera, W. C. Heird, M. Hyde, K. Laitinen, J. Laws, E. L. Daza, I. Lopez-Soldado, M. Makrides, K. F. Michaelsen, S. Olsen, H. Ortega, G. Putet, I. Rogers, P. Roggero, L. Sobotka, H. Szajewska, and H. Weiler. 2007. Dietary fat intakes for pregnant and lactating women. *British Journal of Nutrition* 98(5):873–877.

Lammi-Keefe, C. J. Pregnancy as a risk factor for decreased macular pigment and macular degeneration: Protective potential for DHA/fish consumption. Manuscript in preparation.

Leung, B. M. Y., and B. J. Kaplan. 2009. Perinatal depression: Prevalence, risks, and the nutrition link—A review of the literature. *Journal of the American Dietetic Association* 109(9):1566–1575.

Makrides, M. 2008. Outcomes for mothers and their babies: Do n-3 long-chain polyunsaturated fatty acids and seafoods make a difference? *Journal of the American Dietetic Association* 108(10):1622–1626.

Oken, E., M. L. Østerdal, M. W. Gillman, V. K. Knudsen, T. I. Halldorsson, M. Strøm, D. C. Bellinger, M. Hadders-Algra, K. F. Michaelsen, and S. F. Olsen. 2008. Associations of maternal fish intake during pregnancy and breastfeeding duration with attainment of developmental milestones in early childhood: A study from the Danish National Birth Cohort. *American Journal of Clinical Nutrition* 88(3):789–796.

ANALYSIS OF THE RELATIONSHIP BETWEEN PRENATAL WIC PARTICIPANTS AND BIRTH OUTCOMES

Commenter I

Barbara Devaney, Mathematica Policy Research, Inc.:

> A major limitation with some previous analyses of birth weight is that they did not account for gestational age bias. It is possible to control for gestational age bias by looking at full-term births only. If we know the timing of WIC enrollment or, alternatively, if we restrict the sample to one in which gestational age bias has been removed, then it is possible to estimate the relationship between prenatal WIC participation and birth weight without concern for gestational age bias.
>
> Some argue that there may be limited potential for WIC to affect birth weight. While it is useful to think carefully through a logic model for designing studies of WIC effectiveness, it seems premature to rule out an important line of analysis. The point of a research agenda is to identify research topics of interest, conduct the analysis, and let the results provide the answer, not to dismiss a set of results before doing the analysis.
>
> In summary, given the objectives of the WIC program to address the critical development periods of pregnancy, infancy, and early childhood, a research agenda should include questions related to the effects of prenatal WIC participation on birth outcomes. Rather than reducing the focus on birth outcomes, think carefully about the range of birth outcomes that should be examined. In addition to the important ones identified at the workshop, newborn birth weight should also be considered.

F

Compilation of Proposed Research Topics and Methodological Issues Covered During the Workshop

This appendix contains two major sections: (1) suggested research topics, and (2) suggested methods. The section on research topics is a compilation and condensation of the research topics that were addressed by presenters, discussants, and moderators during the workshop. The topics are organized under themes that emerged during the workshop, some of which differ from the session titles. Suggested research topics that are similar in subject matter have been grouped together even if the suggestions were made during different sessions. The section on methods covers suggestions made by presenters and discussants during sessions one through eight; it does not cover the methodology presentations made during the closing session.

Suggestions differ in style, reflecting differences in the speakers' approach to the assignment. The list does not reflect priorities or group consensus.

PROPOSED RESEARCH TOPICS

Overview

- Additional, more rigorous evaluations of the effectiveness of the Special Supplemental Nutrition Program for Women, Infants, and Children (WIC) (food package, nutrition education, referrals) in:
  - o Improving birth outcomes and reducing health care costs,
  - o Improving diet and diet-related outcomes for mothers and children,

  - Improving infant feeding practices, and
  - Improving inter-natal and prenatal health and nutrition status.
- Effects of the WIC food packages on the dietary behaviors of WIC mothers and young children.
- The effectiveness of prevention and intervention strategies to reduce the risk of overweight and obesity.

Maternal Health and Behaviors

- Observational studies on the effect of interconceptional nutrition on birth outcomes and long-term child health, incorporating biomarkers to identify mechanisms and pathways.
- Nutritional intervention studies that begin during interconception and give priority to women with previous adverse outcomes and communities with marked nutritional health disparities.
- Nutritional research that focuses on women's health before, between, and beyond pregnancies. Inputs to consider include preconceptional smoking, prenatal weight gain, diet, exercise, and smoking cessation. Outcomes to consider include metabolic allostasis and allostatic load, postpartum weight retention, and breastfeeding.
- The impact of coordinated surveillance and communication on the promotion of healthful behaviors during pregnancy and post partum, with the goals of preventing childhood obesity and improving maternal health. The coordination would be among obstetricians and WIC providers (at a minimum); and the targets of intervention would be maternal pre-pregnancy body mass index, excessive gestational weight gain, maternal smoking, and gestational diabetes.
- Interventions associated with the length of gestation.

Breastfeeding

- How to increase breastfeeding rates in the United States.
- Effective strategies for WIC to use to support exclusive breastfeeding and to promote the initiation and duration of breastfeeding. Components of support for breastfeeding include: peer counselor training, roles, contacts, and cultural competency; lactation consultant roles, sufficiency of numbers, and availability; and relationship of counseling to medical care.
- Effects of peer counseling on breastfeeding initiation, exclusivity, and duration; cost-effectiveness.
- Core WIC staffing with regard to the numbers and types of staff members, how they are used, and relationships among them.

- Components of peer counseling implemented by WIC agencies with high-performing programs, prioritizing exclusive breastfeeding and giving attention to ethnic background, race, and acculturation.

Infant and Childhood

New WIC Food Package and Infant Feeding

- New WIC food package for exclusively breastfeeding women: content, presentation, promotion, and implementation.
- The impact of new WIC food packages with regard to breastfeeding initiation, exclusivity, and duration; formula use by partially breastfed infants; and formula feeding.
- The effect of the new infant and child food packages on diet quality and nutritional status, examining the association of meat intake at 6 months with iron status in breastfed infants, and both immediate and longer-term effects of the revised food package.
- The effect of formula feeding on health.

Obesity Prevention

- The effect of WIC participation on growth outcomes using the World Health Organization growth standards (0–24 months), determining outcomes such as the percentages of overweight and underweight infants and effects of the rate of weight gain early in the period on later weight outcomes.
- The effect of coordinated surveillance and communication strategies among WIC providers, home visitation programs, childcare providers, and pediatricians on changing behaviors to help prevent excess weight gain among infants from birth to 12 months. The targets of intervention during infancy would include excess infant weight gain; breastfeeding initiation, continuation, and exclusivity; responsive feeding; portion sizes of bottles and solid food containers; outdoor physical activity; limiting television viewing and televisions in bedrooms; improving sleep quality and duration; coordinated referrals and communication strategies; improvements in parents' ability to handle infant feeding, sleep, and media exposure; and the identification of children at high risk of rapid growth.
- The effects of a coordinated communication strategy among WIC, Head Start, and pediatricians on changing behaviors that help prevent obesity among children 12 to 60 months of age.

- Prospective study of WIC versus non-WIC children, for which outcomes would include body mass index, diet and physical activity, television viewing, and health care utilization. Co-variates to be tracked longitudinally would include the child's family situation, maternal behaviors, Head Start or parenting programs, continuity of care, and neighborhood factors that may contribute to obesity.

Relationships of Food Insecurity with WIC Participation

- Effects of WIC on food insecurity and diet and health outcomes.
- Benefits of different WIC components relative to participants' food security status.
- Relationships of food insecurity with the effectiveness of WIC services in promoting behavior change.
- How WIC can best help families reduce demands and increase capabilities.
- Interactions of WIC with other programs, including the Supplemental Nutrition Assistance Program (SNAP) and Medicaid.
- Program responsiveness to the economic situation.
- Interventions affecting WIC participation, ways to reduce barriers to WIC participation.

Linkages, Collaborative Efforts

- Linkages with other providers (e.g., home visitation, childcare providers, obstetricians/gynecologists, pediatricians).
- Linkages between WIC interventions and health care utilization and outcomes.
- The inclusion of oral health screening, fluoride treatment, dental sealant application, and other basic oral-health activities and referrals as part of WIC services.
- The use of WIC to help establish pediatric medical homes for infant and child participants.

Nutrition Education

- Can WIC nutrition education reduce the risk of obesity?
- Experimental (randomized) trials to compare one method of nutrition education with another (see following section on methods).
- The effectiveness of various modes of delivering nutrition education and the identification of those modes that could be easily adopted at other WIC sites.

- Interventions that increase the consumption of WIC foods by participants.
- Ways in which factors that contribute to health disparities are related to nutrition education.
- WIC's role in providing nutrition education services to postpartum women and to fathers or other caregivers, and to others who influence care.
- The potential applicability of interventions that have been effective in achieving behavior change in settings outside of WIC.
- The durability of the behavioral, consumption, and weight changes achieved among WIC participants with the new WIC package of foods and counseling.
- Methods to make more effective use of technology in WIC's nutrition education activities.

Food Package and Redemption

- Interventions associated with voucher redemption.
- Comparison of food purchases by households that receive WIC vouchers, cash, or SNAP benefits.
- WIC participant purchasing choices and behaviors and factors affecting them, including the accessibility of stores that carry WIC foods and the availability, quality, variety, and cost of WIC foods in those stores.
- Factors affecting the inventories and participation of small stores acting as WIC vendors.
- Ways to make more effective use of technology in WIC, e.g., electric benefit transfer (EBT) machines.
- Ways to further improve the quality of food purchased with WIC vouchers, especially in small urban food stores.
- The use of WIC benefits in farmers markets, community-supported agriculture, and other local and urban food production venues.

Miscellaneous

- Assessment of manufacturer-added functional ingredients as part of the larger process of determining which foods will be allowed in WIC food packages.
- Ways to maintain or increase funds available to WIC.

PROPOSED METHODS

Data

- Link up with surveillance data from the Centers for Disease Control and Prevention (CDC) and make WIC data more publicly available.
- Collect more types of data—not just WIC participation and timing of entry into WIC.
- Use standardized breastfeeding definitions; consider definitions from the Infant Feeding Practices Study II.
- Reduce recall periods to obtain accurate information on the intensity of breastfeeding.
- Collect data on relevant covariates; include prenatal breastfeeding intentions, past breastfeeding history and experience, early hospital experience, reasons for the feeding choice, and the WIC food package chosen.
- Improve the surveillance of obesity-related risk factors.
- Improve the surveillance of infant weight gain using the CDC growth charts.
- Consider ways to improve the accuracy of self-reporting by clients.
- Use focus groups to distinguish characteristics of WIC participants and eligible non-participants.

Selection of Outcomes, Target Behaviors, and Interventions

- Use a logic model to identify appropriate outcomes, target behaviors, and interventions (see Chapter 8).

Examples of Criteria for Target Behaviors

- The behavior has an impact on energy balance or weight, is unlikely to do harm, and has a favorable impact on non-obesity outcomes, such as improving social well-being.
- Consider behaviors that have the highest impacts on obesity prevention, that WIC is in a good position to address, and that are or should be integral to the mission of WIC.
- Target behaviors must matter to partners and caregivers and extend beyond weight and obesity.

Examples of Criteria for Interventions

- Select interventions that are feasible, replicable in many settings, and affordable.

Possible Research Designs

Observations

- Analyze data from the National Health and Nutrition Examination Survey before and after implementation of revised food packages, possibly controlling for characteristics of states' food lists.
- Analyze administrative data from a sample of states.
- Conduct periodic national WIC evaluations to track attitudes and behaviors, food purchasing patterns, the use of vouchers, and the mother–child dyad; allow comparisons across the larger states; track changes in the health of selected WIC women and children over time and compare with changes in a control group.
- Conduct a long-term prospective study of children with differing exposures to WIC (see Chapter 8).
- Compare the dietary intake of those who leave the program with the intake of those who stay, or compare the dietary intakes of early versus late entrants, or both.
- Analyze changes between certification and recertification in such measures as weight status, iron status, and dietary patterns.

Qualitative

- Include a qualitative component to assess participant experiences, identify helpful aspects of the intervention, and mold future processes and policies. Combine qualitative and quantitative formative processes and impact evaluation to assess the effectiveness of new measures.
- Use a multi-stage research design that involves the development and testing of a communication strategy (see Chapter 3).

Experimental

- Compare WIC to an enhanced form of WIC.
- *Randomization by unit, for example, by WIC site or by state* Use an intraclass correlation coefficient to adjust for this type of randomization.
- *Staggered intervention with each unit as its own control* Use an interrupted time series.
- *Delayed treatment design* Start the intervention at one site, compare to another site that does not have the intervention, and then eventually provide it to that site as well.
- Within the WIC population, compare the effects of three delivery approaches: (1) learner-centered (group at clinic), (2) online

learn-at-home (individual), and (3) one-on-one counseling model (control). In each of four to six states with different demographics, select eight clinics: four for approach 1, four for approach 3 (above). Online clients (approach 2) would need to be volunteers recruited from all the study clinics.

- Randomized controlled trial design:
  1. Identify the approaches with which WIC appears to produce an effect (e.g., nutritional advice, smoking cessation).
  2. Offer competitive grants to clinics to improve results along one of the dimensions.
  3. Choose clinics that qualify, and randomly assign some of them to be awarded money and some of them not.

Reporting

- Adopt the Transparent Reporting of Evaluations with Nonrandomized Designs (TREND) statement to allow for a more systematic review of the WIC interventions and possibly for the merging of small datasets,
- Include a strategy statement, which is a description of procedures used in the intervention that is detailed enough that another investigator could replicate the intervention, and
- As part of the research agenda, develop a process for synthesizing and disseminating the WIC research findings.